Horse Care
A Practical Manual of
Horsemastership

Jeremy Houghton Brown
and
Sarah Pilliner

OXFORD

BLACKWELL SCIENTIFIC PUBLICATIONS

LONDON EDINBURGH BOSTON

MELBOURNE PARIS BERLIN VIENNA

© 1994 by Blackwell Scientific Publications
Editorial Offices:
Osney Mead, Oxford OX2 0EL
25 John Street, London WC1N 2BL
23 Ainslie Place, Edinburgh EH3 6AJ
238 Main Street, Cambridge,
  Massachusetts 02142, USA
54 University Street, Carlton,
  Victoria 3053, Australia

Other Editorial Offices:
Librairie Arnette SA
1, rue de Lille
75007 Paris
France

Blackwell Wissenschafts-Verlag GmbH
Kurfürstendamm 57
10707 Berlin
Germany

Blackwell MZV
Feldgasse 13
1238 Wien
Austria

First published 1994

Set by DP Photosetting, Aylesbury, Bucks.
Printed and bound in Great Britain at
the Alden Press Limited, Oxford and
Northampton.

DISTRIBUTORS

Marston Book Services Ltd
PO Box 87
Oxford OX2 0DT
(*Orders:* Tel: 0865 791155
         Fax: 0865 791927
         Telex: 837515)

USA
  Blackwell Scientific Publications, Inc.
  238 Main Street
  Cambridge, MA 02142
  (*Orders:* Tel: 800 759-6102
           617 876 7000)

Canada
  Oxford University Press
  70 Wynford Drive
  Don Mills
  Ontario M3C 1J9
  (*Orders:* Tel: (416) 441-2941)

Australia
  Blackwell Scientific Publications Pty Ltd
  54 University Street
  Carlton, Victoria 3053
  (*Orders:* Tel: 03 347-5552)

British Library
Cataloguing in Publication Data
A Catalogue record for this book is available
from the British Library

ISBN 0–632–03551–X

Library of Congress
Cataloging in Publication Data
Brown, Jeremy Houghton.
    Horse care: the practical manual of
  horsemastership/by Jeremy Houghton
  Brown & Sarah Pilliner.
      p. cm.
    Includes index.
    ISBN 0–632–03551–X (PB)
    1. Horses. I. Pilliner, Sarah. II. Title.
  SF285.3.B765 1994
  636.1'083– –dc20   94-17458
                                          CIP

Contents

Preface

Horse Care: A Practical Manual of Horsemastership, along with *Horse and Stable Management*, brings together for the first time all the information, apart from riding technique, required by those seeking equine National Vocational Qualifications. It is equally appropriate for those taking British Horse Society (BHS), the Association of British Riding Schools (ABRS), the National Pony Society (NPS) or other organizations' examinations, and is very well suited to being a primary textbook for all horse courses at colleges. However, the book is also suitable for the individual horse- or pony-owner who seeks good practice.

The book is divided into three parts. The first part, *Work in the Stable Yard*, starts with handling horses from the ground and then moves on to consider people. In considering people in the stable yard there are sections on supervision, health and safety. The second part of the book, *Horse Care Skills*, is divided into six sections and considers the progressive skills needed for each area. The topics covered include: horse clothing, preparing horses for use, saddlery, feeding and watering, travelling horses and lungeing. The third part, *Horse Care in Action*, shows how the skills become more dynamic, exciting and rewarding as they come together to deliver quality performance.

The titles of the chapters in Parts I and II relate to NVQ units, so those working towards their NVQ will find their progress made easier. Those working at NVQ Level 3 will find that the management of people is dealt with in more depth in the companion volume by J. Houghton Brown and V. Powell-Smith, *Horse Business Management*, Blackwell Scientific Publications.

Horse Care also forms a companion volume to *Horse and Stable Management*, second edition, by J. Houghton Brown and V. Powell-Smith, Blackwell Scientific Publications, which explains in detail how horses work whereas this book is principally concerned with the many skills involved in horse care and working with horses. The book is well illustrated with the majority of photographs supplied by Joanna Prestwich.

The methods described for caring for horses are not the only ones, but they are safe, well proven and generally recommended. The skills shown have been handed down by professionals from a time when horses dominated transport, war and farm work. Over the years they have been refined in the light of new materials, increased veterinary knowledge and higher labour costs. Quality work, attention to detail, pride in turn-out – these are all hallmarks of the horsemaster.

This book will be invaluable to those who are willing to work hard, take pride in their work and are committed to horses.

Jeremy Houghton Brown
Sarah Pilliner

Introduction

Before horses were domesticated they lived in herds ranging over a
wide area. They roamed as they pleased, eating herbage, grasses and
bushes, this wide choice of plants supplying all their nutritional needs.
They drank only once or twice a day because the food they were eating
contained a high percentage of water. In fact they lived much as the
herds of zebra do in Africa today, and one rarely sees a thin zebra!

Man's domestication of the horse has led to the horse being kept

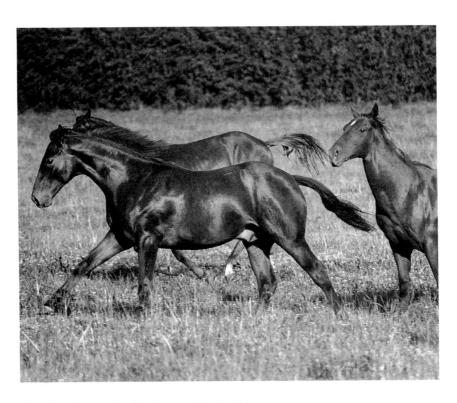

Fig. I.1 Horses evolved as free-ranging herbivores.

captive in paddocks or stables so that we can manipulate its exercise and feeding to suit our own purposes, be it producing a racehorse or a gymkhana pony. With captivity comes a moral responsibility; the horse is entirely dependent on us to provide adequate feed, water and exercise and to provide an environment which will keep the horse healthy. There are also economic considerations; horses are expensive to keep and a healthy, well-kept horse will be better at his job and have fewer costly vet bills.

In order to keep the horse healthy, both in body and in mind, the horsemaster should remember the natural habits of the horse and try to reproduce the same conditions as far as possible. Ideally the horse should be turned out to grass every day and the feeding programme should be arranged so that it covers as wide a period as possible and does not include long periods when food is not available.

The horsemaster's task is to keep the horse fit and healthy in an economical fashion, both in the stable and out at grass. In order to do this the horse must be provided with a clean and safe environment, fed and watered correctly and observed closely so that prompt action can be taken if signs of ill-health are noticed.

Describing the horse

In order to communicate effectively within the horse industry it is necessary to be familiar with a certain amount of 'horsey jargon'; being asked to catch 'the bay mare' may not be very helpful in a field of 20 horses. Describing a horse thoroughly involves identifying the horse's sex, height, colour, markings, age and type.

Sex
The following terms more accurately describe the sex of a horse:

- A *filly* is a female less than four years old.
- A *mare* is a female of four years old or more.
- A *colt* is an uncastrated male of three years old or less.
- As a four year old onwards he is known as a *stallion* or *entire*.
- A *gelding* is a castrated male.

Height
Horses are traditionally measured in hands with one hand being equivalent to four inches. The trend is now for ponies to be measured

Horse measurement in hands and centimetres.

Hands	Centimetres	Hands	Centimetres
11.0	111.6	14.2	147.2
11.2	116.8	15.0	152.4
12.0	121.8	15.2	157.5
12.2	127.0	16.0	162.6
13.0	132.0	16.2	167.6
13.2	137.0	17.0	172.7
14.0	142.2	17.2	177.8

in centimetres as are horses in many other countries, with one hand being equivalent to 10.16 cm. The measurement is taken with the horse standing squarely on a smooth level surface. Measure from the highest point of the withers, using a measuring stick with a spirit level on the cross bar. Take 12 mm (½ in) off the height if the horse is shod.

Colour

The colour and markings of a horse are considered by some people to be significant with tradition suggesting, for example, that chestnut mares are more difficult than mares of other colours. The foal's colour at birth may not indicate the eventual colour with many grey horses, for instance, being born dark. Grey horses also become lighter grey as they get older. Some horses have a summer coat a different shade to their winter coat and may change again when clipped; the colour of the horse's muzzle is used to identify the true colour.

- The *bay* comes in three different shades: the light bay is a golden or reddish brown; the bright bay is a horse-chestnut colour; and the dark bay is a rich dark brown. Bay horses have a black mane, tail and lower leg; these parts of the animal are known as the 'points'.
- The *brown* horse is a darker brown than the dark bay and may appear black until you check the muzzle.
- The *black* horse is black with black points and a black muzzle.
- The *chestnut* also comes in many shades: a liver chestnut verges on brown and tends to have darkish points, but careful examination will show that these are not black; at the other end of the chestnut range comes the lighter chestnut and finally the palomino with its golden body and silvery mane and tail.
- The colour *grey* includes white through to iron grey and the horse

may be dappled to a varying degree. Flea-bitten greys have small flecks of dark hair scattered through the coat.

- A horse is described as *white* if it has a pink skin though more usually the coat is a light cream colour and the eyes may be an unusual bluish colour.
- A *roan* has a mix of white and other colours in the coat giving rise to strawberry (chestnut), red (bay) or blue (diluted black) roans.
- The *dun* may vary from blue, which is a diluted black, to yellow. The mane, tail and lower legs are black and there may be a dark dorsal stripe or 'list' running along the backbone.
- The *piebald* is black and white.
- The *skewbald* is generally brown and white, although it is correctly any colour other than black and white.

This list is not exhaustive and many breed societies have detailed descriptions of allowed colours.

Markings
The horse's markings, including scars, brands and acquired marks from saddle sores, etc., are recorded on veterinary certificates and registration forms.

On the head

- *Star* – a white mark on the forehead. Even if there are only a few hairs, these should be noted.
- *Stripe* – a narrow white mark down the face which may be a continuation of a star when it is described as a star and stripe.
- *Blaze* – a wide covering of white hair running down the face.
- *White face* – an exaggerated blaze covering much of the horse's forehead and face.
- *Snip* – a white mark between the nostrils.
- *White muzzle* – white skin covering both lips and the nostrils.
- *White upper/underlip* – white skin at the edge of the lips.
- *Wall eye* – the eye is a grey–blue colour; sight is not affected.

On the body

- *List, dorsal stripe* or *ray* – the dark line found along the backbone of dun horses and donkeys.
- *Zebra marks* – any stripes found on the body.
- *Whorls* – small areas formed by a change in the direction of hair

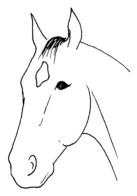

Fig. I.2 Star.

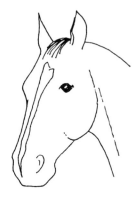

Fig. I.3 Star and stripe.

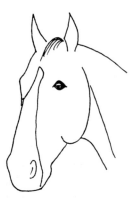

Fig. I.4 Blaze.

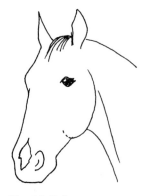

Fig. I.5 Snip.

growth, found, for example, on the forehead and crest of the neck. They are unique to each horse and are in effect the horse's 'fingerprint'.

- *Prophet's thumb mark* – an obvious indentation in the muscle on the neck or shoulder or hindquarters, said to be a sign of good luck.
- *Flesh marks* – patches of pink skin which grow white hair.

The horse may also be marked by scars or brands. Freeze brands resulting in white hair are a method of protecting horses against theft, each horse having its own number and being on a national register. Brands indicating breed or country of origin may be situated on the neck, shoulder or quarters. Identification brands may also be placed on the hooves or tattooed on the lips or gums.

Although not a marking in the traditional sense, it should be noted that horses can also be identified by inserting a microchip about the size of a grain of rice into the neck muscle; it is then reliably identified with a hand-held read-out meter.

On the legs

The terms *white sock, stocking* or *leg* are now only used for casual description and it is more correct to refer to the horse's anatomy. For example, right leg to just below the knee instead of stocking. Black spots on white marks are called *ermine marks*.

Any variation of the colour of the hooves should be noted. Hoof colour usually reflects the colour of the skin on the coronet.

Age

A description of a horse is not complete without including its age. As the biting surface of the incisor (front, cutting) teeth wears away, the pattern on the surface of the tooth changes so that, with experience, the age of the horse can be estimated by examining the teeth. This is described in detail in *Horse and Stable Management*.

Type

A brief description of the type or breed (if known) of the horse is helpful. For example, fine horses are described as light-weight, those with a little more substance are middle-weight and the substantial weight-carrying horse is a heavy-weight. If the breed is not known but the horse has characteristics of a certain breed then it could be described, for example, as a Thoroughbred-type. The idea is to describe the horse in a concise manner, but as clearly as possible

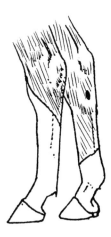

Fig. I.6 White stockings. Left hind: white to lower hock, extending to mid hock. Right hind: white to lower cannon bone.

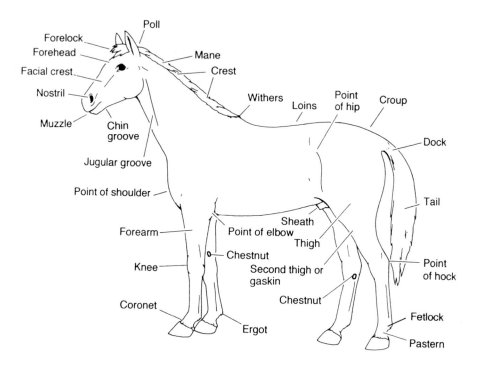

Points of the horse.

Part I
Work in the Stable Yard

1 Handling Horses

Basic handling of horses

Horses are large and potentially dangerous creatures; their natural instincts tell them to flee when danger threatens and if their handler is not aware of this the horse can easily become out of control. As with any other animal, young horses, especially colts, are playful. If not disciplined this 'playing' can get out of hand and the horse becomes wilful and difficult to handle. If not handled with consistent competence and taught good stable manners horses will learn their own strength and use it against their handler, a frightening and dangerous situation. It is essential that, no matter how quiet the horse, the handler always works in a safe manner so that it becomes second nature to do so.

Whenever you are handling horses it is important to try and develop a rapport; use your voice. Horses have very acute hearing so never shout at them. They are also highly sensitive to the tone of voice and can be soothed or reprimanded by the use of subtle changes in the way you speak to them. Fear communicates very rapidly from handler to horse; try to anticipate dangerous situations and always be prepared by having the right equipment and by keeping your wits about you. If a potentially hazardous situation arises try to keep calm, talk quietly to the horse and perhaps stroke or pat him, this will keep your nerves under control as well as his. If you are in doubt about your ability to handle a certain horse or situation always seek help or advice.

Approaching the horse in the stable

Horses have good hearing and are very responsive to the handler's tone of voice. Always speak to the horse when opening the stable door; a horse that is taken by surprise may react violently. If the horse is standing by the door he should stand back as the handler enters. If the horse is standing away from the door the handler should enter the

3

stable, close the door and go up to the horse's shoulder, pat him on the neck and put on a headcollar. If the horse is standing with his head in the corner, making it difficult to approach without passing close to the hindquarters, it may be wise to encourage the horse to come to you.

Putting on a headcollar or halter
Before entering the stable the handler should unfasten the headcollar and uncoil the rope, slipping both safely over one arm. Once the horse has been approached the lead rope should be placed round the horse's neck just below the poll; this is to help control the horse should it try to move away. The cheekpieces of the headcollar should be held in either hand and the noseband slipped round the horse's nose. Then the headpiece should be lifted with the right hand and gently flipped over the horse's poll, catching the end with the left hand which also holds the buckle of the headcollar. Care must be taken not to startle the horse or to let the free end hit the horse in the eye. The buckle should then be secured so that the noseband is two fingers' width below the projecting cheekbone or facial crest and any excess length of headpiece

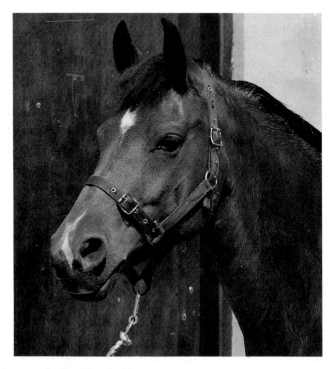

Fig. 1.1 A correctly fitted headcollar.

should be tucked through the headcollar ring out of the way (Fig. 1.1).

Some headcollars are fitted with a browband to prevent the head-piece slipping down the neck. Others have a throatlash secured with a clip and the headcollar is merely slipped over the horse's nose, over the ears and the throatlash is clipped up. The throatlash should be quite loose, allowing a fist between it and the cheekbones. The lead rope should be clipped onto the headcollar under the horse's chin with the open side of the clip under the jaw not the chin and pointing away from it; thus if the horse pulls back he will not catch the fleshy part of the chin in the clip (Fig. 1.2).

Halters consist of rope and incorporate a lead rope. They can be adjusted to fit most horses. However the lead rope must be knotted at the noseband to avoid it tightening on the horse's jaw (Fig. 1.3).

As with all tack, headcollars, halters and lead ropes should be checked regularly and repaired if they are showing signs of wear. Nylon headcollars are not suitable for leaving on horses that are turned out in the field as they do not break should they catch on anything; leather headcollars are safer.

Securing the horse
It is safe practice to tie the horse up when the handler is working in the stable. The horse should be tied with a quick-release knot to a string loop on the tie-up ring (Fig. 1.4). The string loop is designed to break if the horse panics and pulls back. Baling twine is practically unbreakable and should not be used. Horses should never be tied to objects that may move, for example, the stable door or a gate. Mares with foals and untrained young horses should not be tied up.

Horses kept in stalls are tied to a rope which passes through a ring and is then fastened to a sliding log by means of a knot at the end of the rope. As the horse moves in the stall the heavy log takes up the slack of the rope so that there is no danger of the horse putting a leg over a loose rope (Fig. 1.5). Horses may also be cross-tied using two ropes, one from each side of the headcollar, passing to tie-up rings on two posts or two sides of a stall. This is a useful way of keeping the horse still and secure while handling the horse as it limits the range of movement.

The handler must speak when approaching a horse that is tied up to ensure that the horse knows that the handler is there. Do not walk straight up to the horse's bottom and pat him; let him see you and reassure him before touching him.

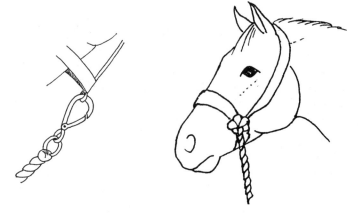

Fig. 1.2 A correctly fitted lead rope clip.

Fig. 1.3 Halter.

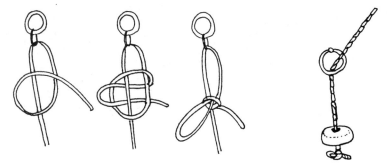

Fig. 1.4 Tying a quick-release knot.

Fig. 1.5 A sliding log and rope arrangement for securing a horse.

Leading a horse in hand off-road

Before taking any horse out of the stable the handler must be sure that they are in control; a quiet, reliable horse can be led in a correctly-fitting, sound headcollar with a lead rope (Fig. 1.6). The handler should be wearing suitable shoes and gloves – nothing hurts like a rope burn – and should never wrap the lead rope around the hand. An overhand knot should be tied in the end of the lead rope. Even so, a naughty horse can quickly learn to pull a short lead rope out of the handler's hands and if there is any doubt about how the horse is going to behave, for example, a young horse or a horse that has been in the stable for a while, the handler should wear a hard hat and lead the horse in a bridle or headcollar with a lunge line attached.

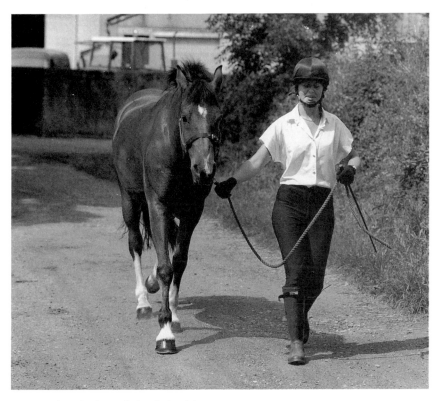

Fig. 1.6 A quiet horse being led safely.

Care must be taken when leading the horse through openings such as stable doors or gateways; do not hurry or take short cuts – the stable door should be open wide and the horse led straight and slowly so that he does not catch his hip. If there is a danger of the gate or door swinging closed on the horse, it should be fastened back or held by a helper; a horse that has had a door or gate swing shut on him may rush, increasing the risk of banging himself or slipping. Once the horse is in the stable, carefully turn him to face the door making sure that he does not slip and then close the door, release the horse and leave the stable.

The horse should be led from the near (left) side with the right hand holding the rope close to the headcollar and the remaining rope coiled in the left hand. The horse should walk freely forwards with the handler at the horse's shoulder. Do not pull on the rope or look back at the horse, if he hangs back either get a helper to encourage him or carry a long whip in the left hand which can be used to tap the hindquarters. (See also Chapter 3, 'The Equine Road Users Code'.)

Presenting a horse for inspection

At some time in his life the horse will have to trot up in hand – it may be for the vet to check soundness or to show the horse off to a potential purchaser – and it is important for both horse and handler to know what they are doing. Ideally there will be a level, straight stretch of hard surface about 40 m long so that there is enough room for the horse to trot forward freely, pull up and turn.

First the horse should be made to stand up straight, square and with his weight equally balanced on all four feet, with the handler standing in front. If the horse is wearing a bridle the reins should be taken over his head and each rein held a little below the bit either side of the head to keep the horse straight and still. When asked, the handler should move to the horse's near side and walk the horse in a straight line away from the examiner until asked to turn. The horse should then be turned to the right, away from the handler, and walked back straight towards the examiner. This is then repeated in trot allowing the horse a few walk strides to balance himself and get straight after turning, before asking him to trot. The horse should not be pulled, held too tight or have his head turned towards the handler as this will prevent the head 'nodding' – the sign of lameness the vet will be looking for.

Turning out into a field

Horses can become quite excited in anticipation of being turned out into a field and the handler must be suitably equipped with gloves, stout shoes and, possibly, a hard hat. The horse should also be suitably restrained. If a normally quiet horse becomes excited and is only wearing a headcollar it can give more control if the rope is placed over the horse's nose from the off side and secured through the noseband of the headcollar. The field gate should be opened wide enough to avoid any risk of the horse banging itself. If there are other horses barging at the gate, help should be sought rather than struggling to squeeze the led horse through and risking injury to horse and handler.

Once the horse is in the field, turn him, close the gate and release him. Horses should never be chased once released. If several horses are being turned out at the same time they should all be led well into the field, turned to face the fence, well apart from each other and released at the same time. The last person in the field closes the gate and tells everybody else when ready to let their horse go. Horses often have a buck and a kick, so turning them to the fence means that they have to turn round to gallop off, giving the handlers a chance to step back out of the way.

Every time a horse is turned out in the field a quick check should be made for hazards such as litter, broken fencing and poisonous plants and action taken as necessary – either clearing up the problem or reporting it to the person in charge.

Catching a horse in the field

Depending on the horse's temperament, catching one horse in a field containing several horses can either be easy or a very frustrating, not to say dangerous, exercise. Go prepared with a suitable headcollar and rope and a few nuts in a bucket if necessary – if there are several horses a bucket can be a liability as they all crowd around to get a mouthful. In this situation the reward may be better hidden in your pocket and just offered to the horse you are trying to catch; this is one situation where giving a horse a titbit is justified.

Having shut the gate, approach the horse's shoulder slowly and quietly with the headcollar discreetly held over your arm or shoulder; do not march straight up to the horse, almost pretend it is not him you are after. Avoid staring at the horse. When you are close, speak to him and offer the food, give him a couple of nuts, a pat and place the rope around his neck before fitting the headcollar. This way you can discourage the horse from moving before you have got the headcollar on.

Quietly lead the horse to the gate, avoiding the other horses, open the gate, lead him through, turn him and close the gate. Assistance may be needed at this point if all the horses decide they want to come with you. Squeezing your horse past may result in him getting caught in the gate or the other horses escaping. If you are on your own scatter some feed on the ground away from the gate to distract the other horses while you lead the caught horse out of the field.

Catching a difficult horse

Some horses are always difficult to catch, while others may become upset by other horses galloping about or by wild, windy weather. Some may let you catch them and then pull away from you; again be prepared and use a headcollar and lunge line or bridle to lead the naughty horse. If possible get help and quietly aim to confine the horse in the corner of the field, with one person either side. Each should carry a headcollar and have some feed for the horse. Never try to herd or chase the horse as it will only make him worse and be very careful that the cornered horse does not spin round and kick out or gallop over the top of you.

Occasionally, leaving the horse, giving him time to settle down and coming back later will work; horses do not like to be ignored. Talking to other horses in the field or catching another horse may excite his curiosity and make him more amenable to being caught because he thinks he is missing out on something! Always assume that youngsters are going to be difficult to catch; this way they are unlikely to get into bad habits.

Simple methods of restraint

It is always safer to have an assistant when treating a horse, trimming or clipping and it is important that the helper is not nervous and is

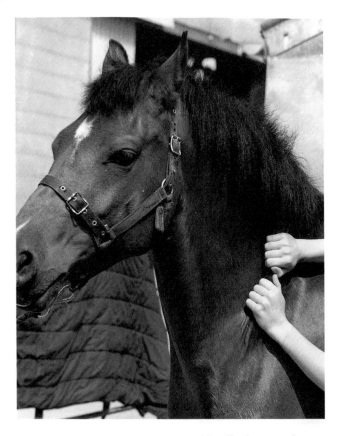

Fig. 1.7 Grasping the skin on the neck can provide effective restraint.

alert, aware and knows what to do. Always start off quietly; a small feed may be enough to distract a horse, or he may respond to being held in a bridle. Do not just put a twitch on the horse with no regard for the horse's temperament.

A simple and gentle restraint is to hold up a horse's front leg; the helper should always be on the same side as the person treating the horse as the horse is more likely to jump away from the treatment than towards it. The horse should be untied and the foot picked up as if the helper is about to pick out the foot and then held by the toe so that the helper can stand upright. Care should be taken that the horse does not snatch the foot away and get a leg over the rope that the helper is holding. If the helper feels about to let go of the foot the other person must be warned so that they can stop what they are doing; remember the other person is relying on the helper for safety.

Grasping a large fold of skin in the middle of the horse's neck is frequently enough to make the horse lower his head and be submissive and is a useful emergency restraint (Fig. 1.7).

Some horses will need more severe restraint and here a twitch is used. A twitch can be made from a piece of broom handle 75–150 cm (2.5–5 ft) long with a piece of stout cord or plaited baling twine looped

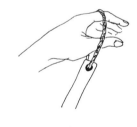

Fig. 1.8 Applying a twitch.

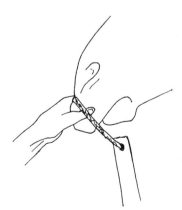

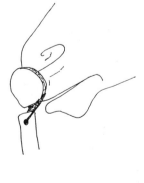

through a hole drilled near the end of the stick. The loop of the twitch is passed over the hand and put on the horse by grasping the upper lip, sliding the loop onto the lip and twisting it tight, adjusting the tension according to the horse's response (Fig. 1.8). The twitch must be put on and taken off quickly or horses will learn to fight it. Most horses react well to the twitch, becoming quiet and amenable. However, a few may try to avoid it, becoming quite dangerous. A sedative or tranquillizer prescribed by the vet may be used for these horses. The horse's ears or tongue should never be twitched and the twitch must not be left on for prolonged periods of time.

Another humane twitch is shaped like a large nutcracker which is passed round the horse's upper lip and then fastened at the open end by a piece of cord. This twitch can be used without an assistant, but this is not recommended because if the horse panics it may be difficult to catch the horse and take the twitch off.

2   The Daily Routine

Yard routine

Routine is as important to those working in the yard as it is to the equine inhabitants; an efficient, yet flexible, routine ensures that all the necessary tasks are completed and gives horses peace of mind. The routine to be followed will vary from yard to yard depending on the type of horse and the priorities of the yard manager. The following routine is rather old-fashioned and would be suitable for hunters or competition horses. Many livery yards would not start until 8 AM while racing yards tend to start earlier.

7.00 AM	*Morning stables*
	Check the horses and refill water buckets
	Tie up, adjust rugs and give haynets
	Muck out
	Quarter
8.00 AM	Feed horses, sweep yard and have breakfast
9.00 AM	Skip out stables
	Tack up and exercise (may be ride and lead)
	On return allow to drink and stale
11.30 AM	Groom and replace rugs. (If there is a second group of horses to exercise, grooming may be done at evening stables)
12.30 PM	Water, hay and give lunch-time feed
	Set fair stable and yard
1.00 PM	Break for lunch
2.00 PM	Carry out daily or weekly chores
	Clean and put away tack

4.00 PM	*Evening stables*
	Tie up, skip out, pick out feet, water and rug up
	Set fair stable, give hay and sweep yard
4.30 PM	Give tea-time feed
7.00 PM	*Late night check*
	Give last feed, water and hay if necessary
	Adjust rugs
	Skip out stables

This routine ensures that the horse's health is checked before he is fed and leaves the horse in peace and quiet to eat his breakfast. However, in many yards the first job of the day is feeding; this is often carried out by a senior member of staff 30 minutes before the rest of the staff arrive. It is important to note and report back whether the horse has eaten all the last night's feed and if there are any signs of ill-health; (the signs of health that should be monitored in an early morning inspection are detailed later in this chapter). Mucking out, tidying the muck heap and sweeping the yard are normally done before breakfast, helping to work up a healthy appetite!

Over breakfast it will be decided which person is to ride which horse and how much exercise the horse needs. Once the horse returns from exercise he is cared for promptly and rugged up again. Many yards try to get all horses ridden in the morning. The horses are then given hay and fed and staff have their lunch break.

The afternoon may be needed for tasks such as clipping and trimming. After the weekly chores any horses not yet fully groomed are attended to and all of the horses are 'done up' for the night. Droppings are picked up from the stables (skipping or skepping out), the banks and the bed are tidied up (setting fair), rugs are changed or straightened, the horses given hay and water and the yard swept. Finally the horses are fed and the yard is locked up for the night. Where possible the horses are given a late night check, water buckets are topped up, rugs straightened and hay and a late feed given if it is in the ration.

On top of the routine outlined above there are other jobs that need to be done. Every day the water buckets and feed mangers must be scrubbed out and automatic drinkers cleaned. Once a week the horses' shoes must be checked so that a shoeing list can be drawn up, the grooming kits should be washed and each horse's rugs shaken out. Yard maintenance routines are described in Chapter 3.

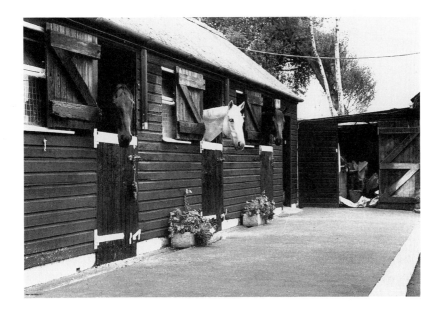

Fig. 2.1 Individual loose boxes.

Choice of stabling

Horses can be housed in different ways depending on factors such as personal preference, cost and the planning authorities.

Individual loose boxes

Loose boxes are the first choice for most horse owners as they allow the horse the freedom to move around and give him his own territory and personal space. However, they can be expensive to build and may be cold and draughty if built in an exposed area. Loose boxes can either stand on their own (Fig. 2.1) or be incorporated into an 'American barn' system where there are rows of loose boxes in a large covered area (Fig. 2.2). This system has several advantages:

- Better working conditions.
- Easier to keep clean and tidy.
- Better security.
- The tack room, feed room and hay store can all be under one roof.

Needless to say there are also disadvantages:

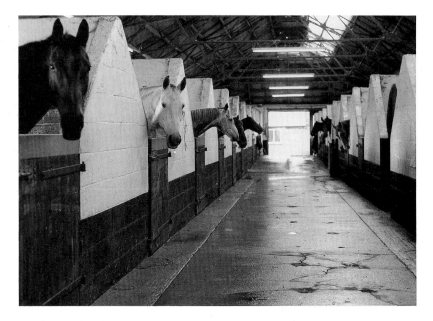

Fig. 2.2 Stabling in an 'American barn' system.

- Fire can spread quickly and it may be difficult to get horses out of the building.
- Ventilation may not be adequate.
- Disease may spread more quickly.

Stalls

Stalls are individually partitioned areas in which the horse is tied up with hay, feed and water placed in front of him. Stalls are also useful as day standings for horses brought in from the field, such as in riding schools. Stalls allow more horses to be housed in a smaller space and are warm, labour-saving, inexpensive and require less bedding material. Mares are particularly easy to muck out in stalls.

Yards

Young horses or riding school ponies may be yarded, in other words several are housed together in a large pen inside a barn. Yards are usually deep littered with straw. Providing that they are watched for bullying at feeding time and no one horse is being 'picked on' this is a natural way to keep horses inside as they are herd animals. In some yards the horses are tethered apart at feeding times.

Beds and bedding

One important aspect of stable management is to provide a clean and safe environment for the horse. This involves 'mucking out', the one job that all grooms are determined not to spend the rest of their lives doing. Mucking out is much like doing the housework – a boring, menial task that is repeated every day while being taken completely for granted by the inhabitants of the house! Yet providing and maintaining suitable bedding is essential to the horse's health and fitness.

A bed is necessary to:

- Prevent injury and encourage the horse to lie down.
- Prevent draughts and keep the horse's lower legs warm.
- Encourage staling and absorb or drain fluid.
- Cushion the feet.
- Keep the horse clean.

Types of bedding material

Ideally the bed should be economical, dry, soft, absorbent of fluid and gases, clean to use, easily obtainable, good quality, not harmful if eaten, light in colour and readily disposable. Few materials can satisfy all these criteria.

Straw

There are three common types of straw which can be used for bedding horses: wheat, barley and oat straw. Generally wheat straw is considered to be the best as it is less palatable to horses and they are less likely to eat it. It is also said to be harder and shorter than the other straws making it easier to handle. However, the horse owner is not always in a position to choose which sort of straw to buy and it is more important that the straw is free from dust and mould. Straw is less absorbent than some other beddings and is best suited to a stable that drains well. Wastage also tends to be greater as it is more difficult to separate clean and dirty straw than, say, clean and dirty shavings.

Straw will rot down and can be spread onto fields as a fertilizer. However, disposal of straw muck heaps is becoming more difficult and European regulations look set to escalate the problems. Although cheap and easily available, straw is not a suitable bedding for horses with a respiratory problem and an alternative should be sought. Dust-extracted chopped straw packed into plastic bags is available; this is more expensive than ordinary straw and may still be eaten by the horse. Hemp straw can also be used; it is highly absorbent.

Wood shavings

Increasing numbers of horses appear to be suffering from respiratory disorders and in an attempt to make the horse's environment as dust-free as possible shavings have become a very popular bedding material. Shavings are compressed and packed into plastic bales and can be bought singly or stored outside, an advantage for the one-horse owner who does not have much storage space. Alternatively the shavings can be bought loose. Shavings are highly absorbent, suiting a poorly drained stable or a deep litter system. Horses are also unlikely to eat shavings making it a very popular bedding for competition horses. One minor disadvantage is that it does tend to get everywhere; rugs need to be shaken out thoroughly and shavings are not a suitable bed for a foaling box. Shavings take a long time to rot down so disposal can be a problem.

Paper

Shredded paper is another dust-free bedding which is highly absorbent. Its use is not so widespread for several reasons: it is expensive, unappealing to the eye and difficult to get rid of. The shreds of paper are very light and tend to blow in the wind so it is useful to put a muck sack over the barrow on the way to the muck heap.

Peat moss

Shavings have largely replaced peat moss which is a dark, dusty and highly absorbent bedding. The dark colour gives the stable a dull look and makes mucking out more of a chore as the droppings and wet patches soon become lost in the bed and regular skipping out is essential. It is very expensive and is sold in plastic-wrapped bales which can be stored outside. It is inedible.

Other materials

The search for economical dust-free bedding continues, with one of the least conventional alternatives being rubber matting covering the stable floor; the matting allows urine to drain away and appears to be comfortable and warm for the horse to lie on as well as being non-slip. As muck disposal becomes more difficult it may be that rubber stable floorings become more popular.

Mucking out equipment

Forks, rakes, shovels and barrows are all potential hazards in a busy stable yard. Observe these guidelines for safety's sake:

- Never leave tools where a horse can reach them and do not put barrows in the stable doorway if the horse is not tied up.
- Store tools out of the way of passing people and animals.
- Do not use tools in need of repair and make sure repairs are safe – string holding something together is not safe.
- During mucking out, prop up outside the stable those tools not in use.
- Move the horse out of the way so that you never have to use the fork close to him.
- Stout footwear is essential as it is only too easy to stab one's foot with the sharp prongs of the fork. Many people wear gloves for protection and hygiene.
- String or plastic from forage or bedding must be disposed of safely in a special bin and not left lying round the yard to cause a hazard.
- Wheelbarrows should be rinsed daily and the remaining tools washed weekly to prevent the muck and urine causing them to rot prematurely.

A three- or four-pronged fork is needed to muck out straw while a special many-pronged fork is used for shavings. Straw beds can be laid with a two-pronged fork. A brush and shovel are needed to tidy up, while all waste is put into a wheelbarrow or muck sack. A skip or skep is a small container used for removing droppings during the day; plastic laundry baskets make an inexpensive skip.

Caring for a straw bed

Ideally the horse should be placed in a separate box while mucking out takes place; this is better for his wind, avoiding the dust that is shaken up during mucking out, and allows more efficient and safe mucking out. If this is not possible, put a headcollar on the horse, tie him to a loop of string on the tie ring and move the horse to one side of the box so that all obvious piles of droppings can be picked up. Remove water buckets and then, starting at the door, use a fork to throw clean straw to the back or one side of the stable. As the straw is shaken the heavier, soiled material falls through the prongs and can be collected on a muck sack or in a wheelbarrow.

Once a week clear and sweep the floor, disinfect it and allow it to dry. The horse should never be asked to stand on bare floor as this is slippery. If the horse has to stay in the box put a thin layer of straw down to stop slipping and yet allow the floor to dry. Regularly turn the banks of straw at the sides of the stable to prevent mould forming; thus throw the bedding to a different side every day.

Then replace the bedding, shaking it well. First build the banks. Banks are useful in preventing draughts and helping to prevent the horse getting cast. Throw the straw up against the wall and then pack it firmly using the back of the fork so that the bank stands above the bed a minimum of 30 cm (12 in) high. Lay the bed so deep that the fork does not strike through to the floor; straw is easily displaced as the horse moves round the box so the bed must be deep enough to ensure that the floor is not exposed – 23–30 cm (9–12 in) should be adequate. Depending on the horse – some are much cleaner than others – allow half a bale of straw per day to keep the bed deep and clean. Large horses in small boxes or brood mares with foals at foot may use as much as a bale a day.

Place the soiled straw on a muck heap, which should be close-packed and neatly squared off. The saying goes that if you want to know if a yard is well run go and look at the muck heap!

Scrub out the water buckets, refill and put back in the stable; do not place them in the doorway or under the haynet or manger, but in a corner where they are visible from the door. If the stable has a fitted manger or drinker check this to make sure that no straw has fallen into it and if necessary clean it out. Both mangers and drinkers should be cleaned daily.

Caring for a shavings bed

The initial cost of laying a shavings bed can be quite high with a 3.7 m^2 (12 ft^2) loose box needing five or six shaving bales to start it off. As before when mucking out, the horse should be taken out of the box or tied up and moved to one side of the box. The piles of droppings can then be picked by hand (wearing rubber gloves) into a skip and then transferred to the barrow. A shavings fork can be used, but, although quicker, this tends to be more wasteful as some clean shavings will be removed. Working from the door the bed can then be thrown up. As the forkful of shavings is thrown against the wall droppings will fall to the bottom of the bank to lie on the floor and can be forked up. As shavings are highly absorbent the wet patches tend to be consolidated like cat litter, not spreading to the rest of the bed. Clean shavings can be scraped off to uncover the wet patches which should then be forked into the barrow.

Once the floor is uncovered it can be swept and, as with straw, either left to dry or have the shavings replaced and new shavings scattered on top. Many shavings are very dusty when fresh and if possible it is better to wait until the horse is out of the box before mucking out. Some people like to put down some clean shavings every day while others put them down a bale at a time when needed. On average two bales of shavings a week should keep the bed topped up adequately, providing that the bed was thick enough in the first place; a foundation of 15 cm (6 in) is the minimum to encourage the horse to lie down and prevent injury.

Deep litter system
Both straw and shavings can be used on a deep litter system. The bed is laid as normal but no droppings or wet patches are taken out. Clean bedding is added whenever necessary. This system is particularly useful when young horses or ponies are yarded together or the stable floor is very uneven or poorly drained. The advantages of the system are that it tends to be economical, less bedding is used on a day-to-day basis, it is labour-saving and provides a solid bed which does not move when the horse rolls.

The system does have some disadvantages: at the end of the winter the bed must be completely removed, often a job for a tractor as it is very heavy work to do by hand; the horse's feet must be regularly picked out; and if the bed is not cared for properly it will become unhygienic and unsightly with the horses covered in muck like cattle. Some yards use a similar system in loose boxes, just taking out the droppings but leaving the wet patches, as outlined in the next section.

Semi-deep litter system
The semi-deep litter system is a useful compromise between a thorough daily mucking out and leaving all the waste in. The way in which yards manage a semi-deep litter system varies from leaving in all the wet material and removing only the droppings daily to removing the wet material and droppings daily but not moving the banks. The latter is a useful way of managing a shavings bed which has very high banks. The banks are left untouched to become quite solid while the middle of the bed is mucked out and the floor swept as normal.

Skipping out

Skipping out involves removing droppings without taking out any bedding. A heavy-duty pair of rubber gloves can be used, particularly in shavings beds. Alternatively a fork can be inserted beneath the dropping and, with the skip tipped towards the dropping, it can be flipped into the skip. The stable should be skipped out every time you go in; this is hygienic and saves bedding from becoming soiled. In any case the stable should be skipped out at lunch-time and evening stables. As long as the stable door is secured and the horse is placid enough it is not necessary to tie the horse up in order to skip out the stable.

Disinfecting boxes

Any stable that has been occupied by a horse suffering from an infectious disease should be thoroughly disinfected before being used by another horse.

- All bedding and left-over hay should be removed and burnt.
- Any salt lick should be thrown away.
- The walls, door, manger and other fittings should first be thoroughly cleaned, possibly with a pressure washer, and then scrubbed with a suitable disinfectant.
- The stable can later be rinsed and left to dry.
- If necessary the walls can then be repainted and the woodwork creosoted.
- Any equipment used on the infected horse or in its stable should also be treated; this includes haynets, grooming kit, buckets, rugs, blankets and tack.

The early morning and late night check

Two important yard routines are the early morning check made before feeding the horses and the late night check made in the evening. The checks are made to ensure that the horse has eaten up its food and looks healthy. In addition the late night check must include a check on the security – everything should be locked and the stable doors secured.

Prompt recognition of the subtle signs of ill-health allows rapid treatment and, consequently, speedy recovery. In order to identify the sick horse the horsemaster must be able to recognize the everyday signs that indicate that the horse is healthy. This should be second nature, a subconscious routine, every time the horse is handled.

The signs of health

- The horse should be alert.
- The horse's stance – it is normal to rest a hind leg, but resting a front leg may indicate problems.
- The horse's mucous membranes (eyelids, gums, etc.) should be a salmon–pink colour.
- The coat should be smooth and glossy, with the skin moving freely over the underlying tissues.
- The frequency, consistency and smell of the droppings and urine should be correct for that horse.
- Disturbed bedding and dried sweat marks may indicate that the horse has been distressed.
- There should be no abnormal heat, pain or swelling on any areas of the horse's body, especially the lower limbs.

If any of these signs are abnormal the first thing to do is to check the horse's vital signs: temperature, pulse rate and respiration rate (TPR). To obtain 'normal' values each of these measurements should be taken while the horse is calm and at rest, for example between feeding and the daily exercise.

Temperature
The horse's normal resting temperature is 38°C (100.5°F). Any deviation from normal may indicate stress of some sort, most commonly illness. A clean veterinary thermometer, lightly greased with petroleum jelly, is used to take a horse's rectal temperature (Fig 2.3). Standing to one side of the horse's hindquarters, lift the tail and gently insert the thermometer into the rectum with a twisting action. Place the thermometer full-length into the rectum, pressing it gently against the wall of the rectum for one to two minutes. Then slowly remove the thermometer with a rotating movement and read it. Digital read-out thermometers, although more expensive, are easy to read and are a useful addition to the first-aid kit.

Pulse
The horse's normal resting pulse rate is 36–42 beats per minute and this corresponds to the heart rate. The easiest place to take the horse's

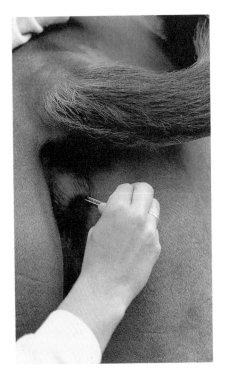

Fig. 2.3 Taking the temperature.

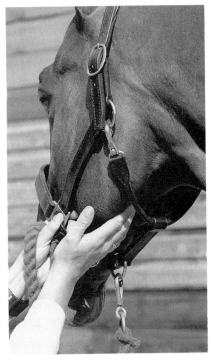

Fig. 2.4 Taking the pulse.

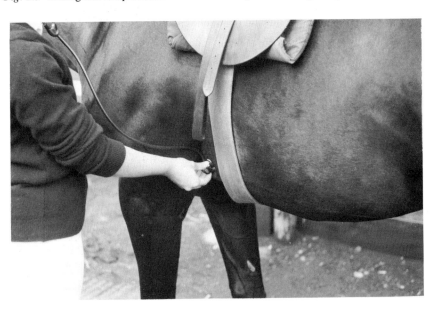

Fig. 2.5 Using a stethoscope.

pulse is where the facial artery runs over the cheekbone (Fig. 2.4). Run the fingers down the inside of the horse's left cheekbone until you feel a moveable lump, about the diameter of a pencil, running across the bone. Gently press your first two fingers along this lump, cupping the cheekbone, and count the pulse for 10 seconds. Multiply by six to give the pulse rate per minute.

A stethoscope can also be used on the left side of the horse, just behind the elbow and in front of the girth (Fig. 2.5). Also, the mounted rider can lean down and press the back of their ungloved hand against the horse in front of the girth. Once the horse has had a canter the heart can be clearly felt hammering against the ribs!

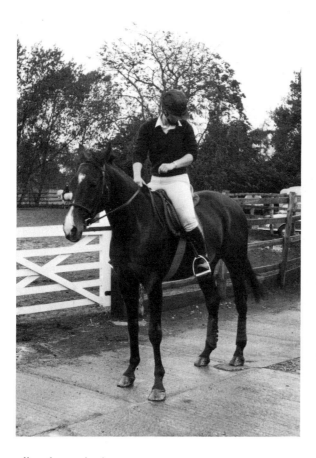

Fig. 2.6 Recording the respiration rate.

Respiration

The horse's normal resting breathing rate – how often the horse breathes in and out – is 8–16 breaths per minute. To take the respiration rate, the in and out motion of the ribs or rise and fall of the flanks is observed (Fig. 2.6). Each combination of in and out is counted as one. The rider can also put a hand close to the horse's nostrils and count as the horse breathes out – beware the horse does not sniff your hand looking for titbits! In cold weather the horse's breath can be seen as he breathes out.

3 Yard Work and Riding Out

Yard maintenance

Safety is paramount; horses are large creatures which evolved to take flight or lash out when threatened and it is essential that anybody involved with horses realizes the potential danger. The yard routine and layout should be organized in such a way as to minimize any risk to the health and safety of both horse and handler. One of the most simple and yet important things is to keep the yard tidy during and after daily chores are carried out. For example, during mucking out tools and barrows should be placed where they will not interfere with the movement of horses and humans, and after use should be stored in a convenient place which is out of the way (Fig. 3.1).

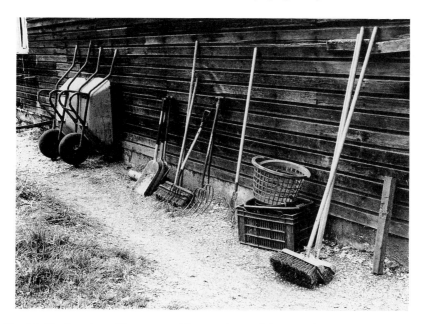

Fig. 3.1 Yard tools and barrows safely stored out of the way.

Disposal of manure

Siting the muck heap
The muck heap should be sited within easy reach of the yard to save
too much time spent wheeling barrows back and forth, yet it should be
out of sight of the car park and yard entrance. The road or track
leading to the muck heap should allow access for the tractor and
trailer or lorry that will remove the manure. The base of the area that
is going to contain the muck should be concreted and surrounded on
three sides by railway sleepers set in steel joists up to a height of 1.8 m
(6 ft). An alternative and time-saving method of muck disposed is to
have a trailer parked below a ramp and to empty the wheelbarrows at
the top of the ramp directly into the trailer which is emptied when full.

Building the muck heap
The muck heap needs daily attention if it is to be kept under control.
The heap should be built in steps with a flat top and vertical sides
which should be raked down to prevent loose pieces of straw blowing
around the yard (Fig. 3.2). The surrounding area must be swept and
kept clean. The secret of success is to pack the soiled straw down as

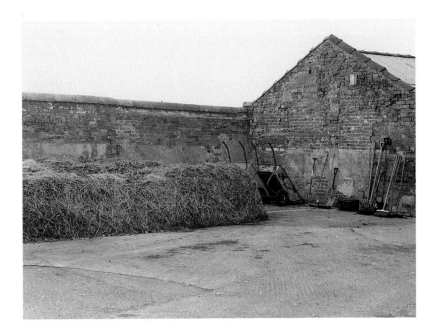

Fig. 3.2 The muck heap.

firmly as possible by stamping it into place; any straw that falls to the floor is thrown up onto the heap and trampled down again. A muck heap built in this way can store more muck in the same area and rots down better because it heats up throughout.

Removing the muck heap

Disposal of manure is a problem for many yards. Straw muck may be regularly collected by firms supplying market gardens and mushroom growers or local farmers may be prepared to spread either shavings or straw muck on their fields. Providing the horses have been regularly and effectively wormed and that the manure is well rotted then the muck may be spread on fields belonging to the yard once or twice a year.

A limited amount of shavings manure may be added to the floor of an indoor school. A muck heap can be burned, but the fire may smoulder for days and sometimes weeks. It can be a fire hazard and may cause considerable nuisance to neighbours.

Weekly chores

As well as keeping the yard and stable area neat and tidy on a day-to-day basis (Fig. 3.3) there are yard maintenance jobs which need to be done on a weekly or seasonal basis. These include:

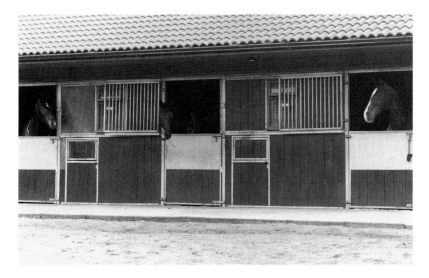

Fig. 3.3 A tidy stable block.

- Cleaning stable windows and removing cobwebs.
- Clearing out drains.
- Checking first-aid kits and fire-fighting equipment.
- Replacing light bulbs.
- Cleaning stored tack.
- Brushing out rugs.
- Cleaning out the feed room, hay and straw shed.
- Scrubbing out feed and water containers.
- Checking feed stocks.
- Ordering and collecting feed.
- Disinfecting stable floors.

Unfortunately many of these jobs are often neglected with staff having more than enough to do caring for the horses. This is short-sighted as maintenance is important for appearance, safety and long life of equipment and fittings.

Clearing drains

Once a week drains and sinks should be flushed with cold water to ensure that they are working properly and then disinfected. Occasionally drains will become blocked and have to be cleared; this unpleasant job should be done with care as there is a health risk involved. Heavy-duty rubber gloves are vital and drainage rods should be used where possible to loosen the material clogging the drain. To prevent some drains blocking they can be fitted with a removable grid or trap which catches solid material and can be cleared regularly. In cold weather drains may freeze over and should be melted with liberal applications of salt.

Disinfecting stable floors

Although desirable, it is unlikely to be feasible to take up the bed once a week, scrub the floor with disinfectant and allow it to dry before putting the bed back down. Thus many yards only do this twice a year and in the meantime sprinkle powdered disinfectant on the swept stable floor once a week. This is a useful compromise which keeps the stable sweet-smelling and is not time consuming.

Personal hygiene

There is little point in maintaining a high standard of stable management if this is not reflected by the staff. Working with horses is a grubby job and yet every effort should be made to maintain personal hygiene: clothing should be clean, hair tied back, fingernails kept short and easy to scrub and no dangling scarfs or jewellery worn which may be unsafe.

Lifting heavy objects

Back pain is the major reason for people being off work, yet lifting heavy and often awkward objects is unavoidable in stable work. Safe procedure will help avoid accidents which often result from careless short cuts (Fig. 3.4). Whenever possible bales and sacks should be moved on a wheelbarrow but they still have to be lifted onto the barrow. To minimize the risk of back injury, any weight should be picked up from the ground by standing in front of it and bending the knees. Avoid lifting a bale or muck sack, swinging it onto your shoulder and turning at the same time; lift it straight up to rest on something and turn before taking hold of it again and carrying it on your shoulder.

Load a barrow with the weight towards the front, over the wheels. Although the temptation is great, avoid overloading barrows, trying to carry too much or moving things single-handed. Full water buckets are easier to carry if the weight is equally distributed so carry one in each hand.

Bales and muck sacks are not the only heavy objects that need to be moved; bags of feed have to moved and stored. Small bags which can be lifted high and held against the chest can generally be carried comfortably, but if you need to lean back to support the weight, the bag is too heavy and should be put on a barrow.

The feed room

The feed room should be conveniently sited to avoid wasting too much time going back and forth to it. It is best constructed of brick or concrete blocks to discourage vermin. It should also be secure so that there is no possibility that a loose horse could stray into the feed room. Large yards may have a feed room and a separate feed shed to allow storage of large quantities of fodder. If this is not the case the feed room should be accessible for door-to-door delivery of feed.

Ideally the room will have a tap, sink and draining board,

- *Assess the situation:*
  Dress – boots, gloves, etc.
  Equipment – pitch fork, bale hook, pulley, trolley, jack, lever, etc.
  Assistance – machine, team, mate, etc.
  Reconnoitre – safe object, safe route, safe landing zone, safe weight.

- *Stance:*
  Feet apart – balanced; one foot forward.
  As close as possible to the object.
  Back straight, chin in.
  Legs bent.

- *Grip (lifting from floor):*
  Hand close and under weight or object clutched close to body.

- *Vision:*
  Do not block your view.

- *Lift:*
  Up and forwards – use leg muscles (calves, thighs, buttocks) but *not* back muscles.
  Do *not* twist or bend your spine.
  Keep weight close to body.

- *Carry:*
  Do not hurry, easy breathing, short steps.

- *Deposit:*
  Reverse of lift.

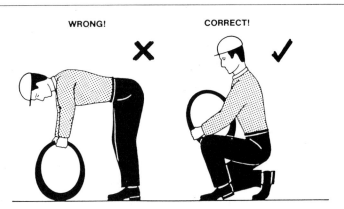

WRONG!   CORRECT!

Fig. 3.4 Safe lifting technique.

encouraging regular washing of feed bowls and utensils. An electric socket for boiling a kettle should be well away from the wet area.

All types of feed will deteriorate if kept in poor conditions; ideally the feed room should be built and designed so that it is always cool with little variation in temperature. It should be well ventilated, dry and light but protected from direct sunlight and free from vermin such as rats, mice, birds, insects and mites.

It is almost impossible to make a feed room vermin proof and so open bags of feed should be stored in galvanized feed bins, raised off the floor on small wooden blocks, or in plastic dustbins with well-fitting lids. These should be cleaned out regularly and always emptied before a new bag of feed is emptied on top. Unopened bags of feed should be stored on pallets to raise them off the ground and prevent dampness. Damp food soon becomes stale, mouldy and unappetizing to horses.

The feed room floor should be swept daily; a commercial type of vacuum cleaner with a long tube will help to keep awkward areas clean. There should be room around the bins for a terrier or cat to patrol and discourage vermin. Empty feed sacks and other rubbish must be collected in a dustbin which should be emptied once a week and any left-over feed should be buried in the muck heap. Simple housekeeping measures like this may not be enough to keep rats and mice away in which case a pest control programme will be needed; rats are a constant health hazard, eating food, making it unpalatable to horses and possibly passing on the disease leptospirosis to horses and dogs. Rats are not the only problem; mice and birds can also rip bags and leave droppings on the floor and in food.

The feed room may also be fitted with a shelf for supplements, a lockable cupboard for medicines and a feed board.

The hay barn and plastic-packed forage

Hay may be stored for daily use in a store in the yard, but large stocks are usually kept in a barn, sited away from the stable because of the fire risk, yet easily accessible to staff. The barn should also be accessible to a tractor for the delivery of hay and straw and there should be no overhead wires which could be damaged by high loads. Even well-made hay loses quality with age, but good storage conditions will help keep it palatable for longer. Hay must be protected from the weather and from damp rising up from the ground. Also air should be able to circulate through the stack so the stack should be raised on pallets or bales of straw and there should be small gaps between the bales. Storing hay in a barn is better than covering it with plastic sheeting as this allows damp and mould to grow – ventilation is very important.

The safety regulations apply to the hay barn as well as the stable yard. String should be knotted and put in a waste bin or bag, any loose hay should be used or cleared up immediately and the bales should not just be taken from the front but removed layer by layer from the top.

Plastic-packed forage will only stay palatable if the bags are not punctured. The bags must be protected from rats and mice which chew the bags and from sharp edges which may rip the bags. Careful handling is also very important. Protecting the bags from direct sunlight will prolong their life.

Monitoring feed stocks

Every week feed stocks should be checked and if necessary ordered or bought. Small yards may visit the local supplier and collect what they require; larger yards may have a weekly or fortnightly delivery. Delivered goods should be checked off against the delivery slip as they are unloaded. This slip should then be checked against the subsequent invoice before paying the bill. It is wise to have an agreement with the feed merchant that if any bags are not up to standard they will be replaced free of charge.

Riding out

When riding out, responsible people know and follow two codes: the Country Code and the Equine Road Users Code (Fig. 3.5).

The Country Code

- Enjoy the countryside and respect its life and work.
- Guard against all risk of fire.
- Fasten all gates.
- Keep dogs under close control.
- Keep to public paths across farm land.
- Use gates to cross fences, hedges and walls.
- Take litter home.
- Help to keep all water clean.
- Protect wildlife, plants and trees.
- Make no unnecessary noise.

Remember that you have a responsibility to yourself, your horse, the

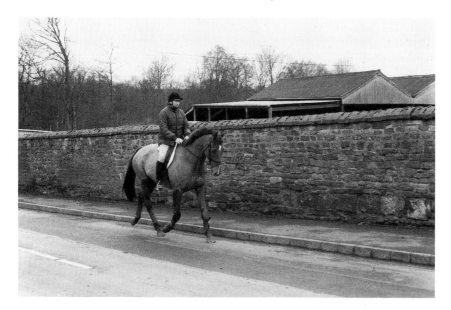

Fig. 3.5 Riding out safely dressed and equipped.

land, farmers and other path users. Behaviour which spoils other people's pleasure, causes accidents, damages crops or stock or inconveniences landowners leads to barred gates and a 'horses not welcome' attitude.

The Equine Road Users Code

- Untrained horses or inexperienced riders may not go on the road alone, nor may they go on busy highways until the rider is experienced and the horse well behaved on quieter roads.
- Riders and drivers must be familiar with the Highway Code and the British Horse Society publication *Riding Safely on the Roads.*
- Horses must stay on the left. Led horses should be on the left of their leader.
- Horses may not go on pavements.
- Riders must wear fitted, properly secured hats to current BSI specifications.
- Footwear must have heels, soles should not have heavy cleats and stirrups must be wide enough.
- Tack must be in good order and properly fitted.
- Bright wear is advisable and in poor light it is essential on both

horse and rider. After sunset a lamp (white – front, red – rear) is required.

- Respect other road users and adjacent pedestrians.

4   People in the Stable Yard

There has been a natural tendency for people involved in working with horses and yard management to concentrate on the horses. They are concerned about the stables, the bedding, the feed, the exercise and so on, but they rarely ask 'Are the staff all right?'. This chapter is about people. If the people are not right then the horses will be unhappy, poorly cared for and unsuccessful.

There was a time when 'girl grooms were two a penny', or so some people seemed to think. There seemed to be enough stable staff so devoted to the needs of the horses in their care that they would work all hours for very little money, living in terrible conditions and getting rare appreciation and few thanks. Mercifully, times have changed and there is now an awareness that staff deserve a square deal and good staff are a sound investment. Furthermore, it makes sense for a horse business to invest in people. Yards that offer fair conditions of service plus staff training tend to keep their staff and have successful results.

Yard staff

Work with horses seems attractive from a distance – cuddling those noble creatures and galloping about with one's hair blowing in the breeze! In reality it is tough, dirty and repetitive. It sometimes calls for courage and a cool approach to tense situations. It requires great pride in one's work, good attention to detail and resourcefulness. Also the person must have that quality of empathy with horses, which in a non-sentimental way creates a good working relationship with them.

What makes a really good worker? The following qualities give some useful pointers:

- *Responsibility* – taking responsibility means that the horse, other people in the yard and all concerned can be quietly confident that each job will be done properly. A person can only work to the best of their ability, but that does include taking pride and interest in the work. Nowadays people rarely have to do a job just because someone says so. They like to understand why the job is necessary and why they do it in a particular way; then personal pride ensures that not only will the job be well done but that everybody can rely on the person to do it.

- *Reliability* – being reliable means that not only can someone rely on the person to do the job but also that it will be done in the agreed manner and at the agreed time. If it is not possible to achieve the plan then the reliable worker will always let the appropriate person know so that a contingency arrangement can be made.

- *Efficiency* – using time efficiently does not mean dashing about, puffing and blowing, driving everyone else to despair and turning the horses into nervous wrecks. It means being well prepared, thinking first and making a plan. Someone who uses time efficiently is also punctual. This does not mean always being early, but it does mean that if the horses have to be loaded at 8.30 AM then by 8.25 AM they are all ready and that one can enjoy the five minutes in hand to mentally check that everything is in its right place according to plan. Sometimes in the horse world this aspect of leaving on time means an early start. The alternative is tasks done badly, the horses flustered and then having a horrid journey because the driver is going too fast for their comfort.

- *Skill* – being skilled means that one has taken the trouble to study how jobs should be done. Then with the aid of good tuition backed up by careful practice the skill is developed, first to a high standard and then to a fair speed. With horses and ponies there is always the extra dimension that the worker must consider the animal and work accordingly.

- *Realism* – each person has to recognize their own limitations and present skill levels. Perfection is usually an impossible dream. Once a person recognizes these things then they can work to improve their knowledge and skills.

- *Resourcefulness* – initiative is a great gift and sadly some people have only a short supply. Working with horses means that nothing is predictable. All animals and much of nature have this factor which makes them so intriguing. One has to cope to the best of one's ability with this unpredictableness. A person must also be willing to say if they do not understand or they need assistance or guidance about how best to proceed. There will also be times when a person finds that their knowledge and skills are not sufficient; in these situations it is generally best to get expert help. It is wrong to feel that one always has to find a solution to every situation independently.

- *Safety* – safe is good. Taking unnecessary risks is bad. Never attempt makeshift repairs – they will let someone down. Try not to skimp jobs by taking short cuts; agreed practice is safe practice. Some people seem accident-prone and disaster seems to follow them around. Watch such people and see why things go wrong. Generally they do not allow enough time; then they fail to engage the brain before starting on the job. It is very important that a person working in the yard does not put others at risk.

For example, there is a dark corridor and you switch on the light; 'pop' – the light bulb blows. It is essential that the bulb is replaced before someone has an accident wandering along in the dark. You put down a rake the wrong way round and someone steps on it; 'bang' – they get hit in the face. You are carrying a bucket and rush to answer the phone; 'crash' – someone has tripped over the bucket. You park your wheelbarrow in the stable doorway because you are late and to save tying up the horse; 'crash, scrape, clatter' – the horse has tried to hop over the barrow or squeeze past it, has fallen in the process and now needs the vet. You open the door of the indoor school; 'crunch, – someone was riding past. You are lungeing a quiet horse without wearing gloves; 'bang' – the farmer over the hedge shoots at a pigeon, your horse leaps in fright and your hands get a nasty burn from the lunge line. The list is endless. All too often accidents do not happen, they are caused.

- *Care* – equine welfare is a concern of every animal lover. Because they are working with horses routinely, some people occasionally lose sight of the animals' needs, or they fail to recognize that each horse is different with individual needs. One must care for the horses' physical and mental well-being.

In competition there is a delicate balance: the event rider or long-distance rider knows that their team-mates and maybe their country depends on them but their horse is exhausted. The prize is within sight – should they press on? No. One must realize that it is fine to stress a horse in competition but he must not be over-stressed. The balance calls for fine judgement, but if there is doubt then the balance must tip towards the horse's well-being rather than competition success.

In riding and driving there is a risk for both horse and handler; riding is a risk sport. However, one must never lose sight of the welfare considerations. Furthermore, at any time or place where one sees unacceptable standards of horse care or misuse of horses one must be prepared to act. The animals which give us so much are owed this.

- *Loyalty* – loyalty is an important quality and takes many forms. A person is loyal in support of their horses and workmates. It is also important to be loyal to the yard and the business; this may entail keeping confidences. During World War II there were posters reminding people that 'Careless talk costs lives' – enemy spies were about. Nowadays one would do well to remember that careless talk costs reputations. Sadly some horse people delight in speaking ill of others.

- *Representativeness* – a final quality of a good worker is that of an ambassador. Everyone is an ambassador, firstly representing themselves, their appearance and pleasant manner immediately establishing a good first impression. Remember, 'You never get a second chance to make a first impression'. One also represents one's team of workmates – one scruffy or loudmouthed person in the team stands out and lets the side down. In addition one is an ambassador for the stable and every stable needs a good reputation. It is a great honour to work for an establishment that is held in high regard. Professionals find that having worked at a yard with a good reputation will always stand them in good stead for the rest of their career.

Working relationships

For most stable staff it is important that they have good relationships with others. Single-handed jobs need a special, strongly-motivated person who can take pleasure from working alone. But most stable yards rely on a team approach and that needs some extra qualities to those already listed.

Everyone in a yard needs to 'pull their weight'. If one person is a slacker then everyone else has to work harder or else standards fall. Also each person must contribute positively to a team approach; some people take the attitude that it is always someone else's job to greet a stranger, pick up litter, change a light bulb or do any other task. The other crucial ingredient for a good team worker is that they promote good relationships and have a good effect on the rest of the team. Everyone has 'off' days when workmates find the person grumpy or a bit difficult; there is generally a good reason. On these days the rest of the team will make allowances. Similarly, there will be times when one is relied upon by workmates.

Maintaining good working relationships with others is important and should not be taken for granted. Working as a team is enjoyable and, if well done, aids efficiency. It is important to be able to take orders and deal with requests; some people all too easily take offence when none is intended. If it is something which cannot be done now then it is helpful to clearly and politely say so. If a problem crops up between one person and another it is important to try and talk it through and resolve it; if necessary a senior person may be brought in to help. The great thing is that the team should be strong and harmonious.

There is a golden rule for being a member of a team: it comes from the Bible in the Sermon on the Mount – 'In everything, do unto others as you would have them do unto you.'

Meeting and greeting

One of the first tasks anyone in the yard must master is how to greet callers. The person may be a client, a potential burglar, have got lost or is just being nosey. A stranger wandering around is an accident risk, and every yard should have an agreed procedure for visitors. Usually there will be an area where they can be 'parked' while the person they need to see is located. A conversation with a stranger in the yard may go like this:

'Good morning. May I help you?'
'No thanks. I'm fine.'
'We have a policy in this yard that no visitor may proceed unescorted. Now, how may I help you?'
'I want to see the boss.'
'I am sorry but Mr Jones is not here at present. Would you like to see the Head Girl?'

Politeness and firmness are the best policy. Anyone without a convincing explanation should have their car registration number and a brief description of their appearance noted in the day book. Then if there is a break-in in the vicinity inform the police. However, never lose sight of the possibility that an unexpected stranger may be a journalist about to write-up your yard in the local paper, or they may be a newcomer to the district seeking to place a lot of business with your yard. Remember too that every message is important. There must be a good system for passing on messages accurately, speedily and reliably.

Supervisory skills

The job of the Head Girl, Senior Lad, supervisor, or whatever title is used, is crucial to the atmosphere of the yard, the level of horse care, tidiness and much else besides.

A good supervisor is easily identified by two particular aspects of the yard:

- Good practice – for every yard there must be selected and agreed safe, effective and efficient ways of doing all routine tasks. All staff including trainees must adopt and stick to these practices. The supervisor is the arbiter of good practice.
- High standards – standards of quality, tidiness and, where appropriate, of work rate are consistently high. The supervisor leads from the front with a forthright cheery example.

A good supervisor has two particular attributes:

- Reliability – reliability is not just necessary from the employer's point of view; it is also sought by all team members. A good supervisor will always do their best, both for the employer and for the staff; where their needs conflict the supervisor may seek a compromise but ultimately has to enforce the employer's requirements with tact, loyalty and authority – it is sometimes a tough job.
- Skill – change must be brought in with understanding, clarity and ongoing enforcement. The supervisor should use their authority without giving rise to resentment. Problems should be dealt with clearly but pleasantly, be they problems with jobs, people or horses. The supervisor advises, demonstrates, refers and helps both individuals and teams in order to achieve high performance. Yet after listening to and discussing others' ideas the supervisor

should always be willing to accept improvements. This person should be a good communicator; they should accept that a good relationship with the team is a two-way process and show authority and sensitivity in making it good.

A particularly difficult skill is that of counselling. Staff have problems and may seek help. The skill lies in listening and then helping the person to reflect wisely on possible alternative scenarios. The mistake is to give pat solutions or trite advice for others' problems. Where appropriate it may be best to tactfully encourage staff towards suitable help from specialists.

Staff training

The yard supervisor together with the employer will design the staff training programme, basing it on an assessment of each person's needs and ambitions. As training proceeds each individual will be given the opportunity to report on their own perception of their progress and how this affects their training plan. The supervisor will review the effectiveness of the training methods being used.

Often the supervisor is the trainer, so they will plan and deliver the training. Staff will need encouragement and will want to know how well they are progressing. The employer will also want to know how beneficial the training is proving to be.

In many cases National Vocational Qualifications (NVQs) will be used which means that staff will have plenty of ongoing feedback on their level of skills and on their progress. British Horse Society qualifications, or those of other organizations, may also be used in parallel with NVQs.

The supervisor has to develop as an effective trainer and so will need training themself to be skilled and up-to-date on qualifications, training techniques and resources.

5   Health and Safety

In Britain there is a Health and Safety Executive which gives advice on good practice and which enforces the relevant laws. People working with horses should know what the law has to say, in general terms, about matters which affect them in their work.

The points below are set out in the Health and Safety at Work Act 1972, a shortened copy of which has to be on display or given to each employee. The Management of Health and Safety at Work Regulations 1992 requires employers to assess risks to staff and others so that risks are minimized; this should lead to proper staff training and supervision to ensure that agreed procedures are followed. The law also requires that records are kept, staff are trained, safety equipment is tested, accidents and incidents are recorded, safety clothing is used where appropriate and dangerous substances are properly stored and used.

Duties of employers

The employer must make reasonably sure that the workplace, all machinery and systems of work are safe. All the kit and anything used must be safe and handled, stored and moved about safely. The employer must make sure that all staff are taught how to do jobs safely and that they are supervized so that they adhere to safe practices. There must also be provision for welfare, such as a first-aid kit, lavatories, hand-washing facilities and somewhere to get warm after working outside in winter.

Duties of staff

Staff, including trainees, must cooperate on safety and health matters. Staff must also take reasonable care for themselves, their workmates and anyone else who may be affected by what they do or fail to do. Those who are self-employed are both employer and staff all rolled into one and so must take on the responsibilities of both.

Safety policy and records

If there are five or more staff the employer has to write a safety policy which staff must be familiar with and obey.

Reporting incidents

Staff should always report incidents when things go wrong. The person in charge can then decide if the matter should be entered in the accident or incident book. Such a book is compulsory for BHS and ABRS approved riding schools; it is also required by the 1981 First Aid Regulations. The entry must show the time, date and place of the incident; it must include the names and addresses of witnesses; it must give a clear account of what happened; it must include the names of the horses and people involved and state who was in charge and who was hurt, with added details of any injury sustained and treatment given; it should include a plan or diagram of the accident, plus informative notes, clearly written, and be signed by both the person in charge and, if possible, the person who suffered the incident. If a loose leaf form is used it should be kept in a file with an index of contents.

Reporting hazards

Any machinery or equipment which is faulty or anything hazardous must be reported to the person in charge as soon as it is noticed. That person has a duty to act straight away. A simple notice stating 'Faulty – do not use' could be the first step, or 'Slippery surface – take care'; then further steps must be taken to put the matter right.

Reporting injuries, diseases and dangerous occurrences

Certain matters have to be reported to the local environmental health department; this is enforced by the Reporting of Injuries, Diseases and Dangerous Occurrences Regulations (RIDDOR) 1985. These matters have to be reported immediately by telephone and then confirmed in writing; the yard has to keep its own record for at least three years.

Examples of injuries which must be reported include:

- Death in an accident at work.

- When a member of staff is off work for more than three days following an accident at work.
- Most broken bones (but not fingers and toes).
- Eye wounds.
- Amputations.
- Injury or unconsciousness from electric shock or lack of oxygen or due to absorption of a substance through breathing, eating or drinking it or from having it spilt on the skin.
- Acute illness from bacteria or fungi or other infected material.
- Any injury which results in the person being admitted to hospital for more than 24 hours; this includes clients at riding establishments.

'Dangerous occurrences' which have to be reported are more likely to occur in factories or on building sites.

Reportable diseases include:

- Asthma caused by working in consistently dusty conditions.
- 'Farmers Lung' which is a breathing difficulty caused by regularly handling mouldy hay or straw.
- Leptospirosis (Weils disease) which can be contracted when working in places infested by rats.

First aid

Under the Health and Safety (First Aid) Regulations 1981 the yard must have first-aid provision. This means that someone must always be in charge and take responsibility for calling an ambulance if it is needed. Ideally this person should have first-aid training. First-aid boxes and kits should be kept at the stables, in vehicles and taken on expeditions.

Accident procedures (when a person is badly hurt)

Accidents can and will occur; frequently they involve a rider falling from a horse on the road, in the school or in a field. Whatever the cause the procedure to follow is much the same. Most importantly remember to *keep calm* and use your *commonsense*. The telephone number of your local doctor and vet should be beside the telephone or carried with you on a hack. Remember that a telephone is no good locked in the house; yard staff must always have access to one. A small emergency first-aid pack must be taken with you on a hack, along with money or a phone card.

Immediately after the accident has happened, secure the scene in order to minimize the risk to yourself and any others in the vicinity. Do this by standing guard over the hurt person while sending others to catch the loose horse and to summon the police and/or ambulance if appropriate. The first priority is the casualty who should be reassured and examined. Be sure to take no unnecessary risks. The next thing is to remember the accident ABC:

- A is for approach and airway. Approach the hurt person being careful not to get hurt yourself, and once you have reached them ensure that their mouth and windpipe are free of obstruction.
- B is for breathing; mouth-to-mouth resuscitation may be necessary.
- C is for circulation; if the person is bleeding, pressure must be applied to the area to stop the bleeding as rapidly as possible.

Check for consciousness

Speak loudly and clearly to the casualty, watching the eyes to see if they flicker or open. If the person is conscious they should be asked if they have any pain in the back or neck and if the answer is 'yes' they must not be moved and you should stay with them until help arrives.

Open the airway

The unconscious casualty's airway may be blocked making breathing difficult or impossible. It is vital to, firstly, remove any obvious obstruction from the mouth and, secondly, to open the airway. This is done by placing two fingers under the chin to lift the jaw. At the same time the head should be tilted well back. If a head or neck injury is suspected the head should only be tilted just enough to open the airway.

Check for breathing and a pulse

Look for chest movements, listen for the sound of breathing and feel for breath on your cheek. The pulse can be felt on the neck, between the Adam's apple and the strap muscle that runs across the neck to the breastbone.

The recovery position and mouth-to-mouth resuscitation
If skilled help is not going to arrive quickly the casualty can be put in
the recovery position. This prevents the tongue from blocking the
throat and allows the unconscious casualty to be left if necessary. It
involves turning the casualty with minimum movement of the head,
neck and spine. In order to turn an injured person without help:

(1) Open the airway.
(2) Straighten the legs.
(3) Kneeling at the person's side, bring the arm nearest you out at
     right-angles to their body, with the elbow bent and the hand
     palm uppermost.
(4) Bring the other arm across the chest and hold the hand, palm
     outwards, against the casualty's cheek.
(5) With the other hand grasp the thigh furthest away and pull the
     knee up, keeping the foot flat on the ground.
(6) Keeping the hand pressed against the cheek, pull at the thigh to
     roll the person gently towards you, supporting the head all the
     time.
(7) Once the person is turned, tilt the head to make sure the airway is
     open and adjust the hand under the cheek to ensure that it stays
     open.
(8) Bend and bring forward the upper knee to prevent further
     movement.

In serious cases the casualty may be unconscious and not breathing.
Immediate action must be taken:

● Undo the chin strap of the hat, but leave it on.
● Press back on the person's forehead and lift the jaw up and
  forwards to open the air passage to the lungs.
● If this does not start their breathing support the jaw, pinch the
  nose and blow a normal breath into their mouth, repeating every
  five seconds.
● Watch to see if the chest begins to rise and fall; if not check that the
  airway is not still obstructed.
● A Laerdal pocket mask is available to avoid the risk of trans-
  mission of disease from mouth-to-mouth resuscitation.

Even if the fallen rider appears to be unhurt, if there is any doubt call
for medical assistance or send the person to hospital for a check-up

and remember to fill in an accident report no matter how minor the incident. Anyone who has, or might have been, concussed must not ride or drive again that day.

Control of Substances Hazardous to Health (COSHH) Regulations 1988

The COSHH Regulations require the employer to make sure that exposure to hazardous substances is prevented or adequately controlled. Such substances include those that are toxic, harmful, irritant or corrosive. They include disinfectants, detergents, insecticides, mouse and rat poison, creosote and veterinary products. The Regulations also cover exposure to harmful micro-organisms such as those which cause tetanus and to quantities of dust from feed, bedding or arenas, or exposure to any material at work which can harm health.

Precautions

The employer must list the hazards, assess the risks, introduce appropriate controls, ensure that these control measures are adhered to and monitor, train and supervise staff concerning risks and precautions. Some matters call for education and training; for example, staff should know that toilet cleaner and bleach are hazardous when mixed; weedkillers should not be decanted into smaller containers as only the original container will be labelled safely.

Sometimes a change of practice is called for, for example, the sump-oil used for horses' feet can give grooms acne. Other matters may call for expensive equipment, for example, riding arenas should not be excessively dusty and need to be kept damp, perhaps requiring an irrigation system. Inexpensive equipment may be needed such as simple dust masks for those grooming muddy horses or stacking old straw. Precautions may involve providing equipment and giving training, such as in the use of rubber gloves, aprons and boots when handling horses with ringworm.

Some of the simple precautions call for an absolute insistence on basic hygiene. Waterproof plasters should cover cuts and hands should be washed before eating (or smoking!). These simple measures reduce the risk of leptospirosis following handling of straw which has had contact with rats. Everyone working with horses should be vaccinated against tetanus.

Safe storage

All pesticides must be stored in a safe lock-up away from staff and feeds. Agricultural pesticides may only be used by staff who have been trained and certified as competent. Veterinary products should be kept in a locked cabinet; only those with adequate training should use these products. If a syringe and needle are used then the needle must be disposed of into a 'sharps bin' – generally found in the back of the vet's car.

Accident prevention

Good housekeeping reduces trips and falls. Pot holes, broken steps, defective gates, projecting nails, items left in passages, tools lying about and any obstruction can cause an accident. Children should not roam unsupervised around work areas.

Those riding or leading horses on the road should keep to the left and the horse should be on the handler's left. Both horse and handler should be properly trained and equipped; inexperienced or overfresh horses should be escorted by a car.

Approved hard hats must be properly fitted and fastened before mounting and remain so until dismounting. Footwear for riding must have a sharp-edged heel (trainers or Wellington boots must never be worn). Footwear for stable work should be robust and, when handling young horses, toe protection is advisable. Gloves should be worn for lungeing and leading young and fresh horses. Bridles give greater restraint than a headcollar.

All electrical appliances and extension cables should be connected using a safety cut-out (residual current device or RCD). Tractors, and even lawn mowers, must only be used by trained staff, as should chaff cutters and oat rollers which must be guarded. Horse walkers should be in a fenced-off area and staff trained before using them. Pressure washers combine water and electricity so need special care. The use of ladders requires caution: the base must not slip so it may need securing on a shiny floor; the top must be at least 1.05 m (3 ft 6 in) above the landing place. If a ladder is left in place, a board must be tied to it so children cannot climb up. Agreed procedures must be implemented when entering riding schools. Finally it is best to keep visitors and traffic away from horses. Wandering visitors should always be greeted and escorted to a safe place. Safety is everyone's responsibility.

Part II
Horse Care Skills

6 Care of Tack and Horse Clothing

Apart from the tack in which the horse is ridden, the domesticated horse wears rugs, blankets and sheets, bandages and boots.

Care of tack

The majority of a horse's tack is made of leather and both leather and stitching will rot if exposed to sweat, water, heat and then neglected. Thus it is important for appearance, safety and durability that it is kept clean and supple. It is also an ideal time to check the stitching and leather for signs of wear and damage. Unsafe tack should be put to one side and not used again until it is mended, otherwise it may break and cause an accident. The stitching on stirrup leathers tends to wear relatively quickly. To check it, grasp the sewn-down end and pull firmly; if the stitching is weak it will be possible to tear the end away. Remember, tack that has broken and been repaired, for example reins, are weakened and should not be used for competition or other strong work.

Many yards only clean the bit and wipe the tack over on a daily basis, just removing straps from their keepers to clean and soap underneath. If this is the case the tack should be taken apart and cleaned thoroughly once a week. If the tack is exposed to much mud and rain then it should be treated with a leather dressing such as neat's-foot oil on a monthly basis. Over-oiling will make reins difficult to hold and may rot the stitching. The stirrup leathers and surface of the saddle should be treated with care or the leather dressing will come off onto the rider's clothing. Similarly, if a saddle is used without a numnah, leather dressing used on the lining of the saddle may stain the horse's back or cause a reaction on a sensitive horse.

Leatherwork should be rubbed clean with a damp cloth or sponge which is regularly rinsed in warm water. Saddle soap should then be rubbed well into the leather, particularly the fleshy or rough side, using a slightly damp sponge. Saddle soap comes in many forms: glycerine, tins, tubes and liquid. Read the instructions and remember not to use too much or to make the sponge too damp.

Only if the tack is caked with mud is it necessary to use more water and get the tack really wet. Wet leather should be dried with a chamois leather or dry cloth. If the leather has been soaked with rain it should be wiped clean and left to dry naturally. A suitable leather dressing or oil should be used before the leather is soaped to replace the oils lost and to prevent the leather drying out and becoming brittle.

Leather may become mouldy or dry during storage. This can be prevented by dismantling the piece of tack, treating it with a leather dressing, wrapping it in newspaper and then putting it in a plastic bag.

Cleaning saddles

The saddle should be placed on a saddle horse and the girth, leathers, irons and numnah removed. If the irons and stirrup treads are very dirty they can be taken off the leathers, separated and dunked in warm water in a bucket. First the underneath of the saddle should be wiped with a damp cloth or sponge, a clean stable rubber put on the saddle horse and the saddle replaced.

The rest of the saddle should be cleaned, removing any lumps of accumulated grease (jockeys) with a pad of horsehair. The seat of the saddle may not need wiping if it is clean. The leathers, girth, irons and treads should be washed, paying particular attention to any folded areas. All the leather should then be soaped, taking care to do both sides of buckle guards and girth straps. The seat and saddle flaps should be wiped with a dry cloth to remove excess soap which may stain the rider's breeches. Irons and treads should be dried with a towel and polished if necessary. Any suede, serge or linen surfaces should not be soaped but brushed clean. After cleaning the leathers, the irons should be replaced, run up and the leathers put through and under the irons. The girth can be laid on top of the saddle and the saddle covered with a cloth or cover before being returned to its rack.

Cleaning girths

Leather girths should be carefully cleaned after use or they will become hard and rub the horse. The inner felt lining of three-fold girths should be removed, oiled and replaced regularly.

Nylon, string, lampwick and webbing girths should be brushed off every time they are used. If they are muddy or stained they should be soaked in a non-biological detergent, scrubbed and thoroughly rinsed. Care must be taken not to soak any leather parts and if they are hung up by both buckle ends to dry this will prevent the buckles rusting. Finally, any leather parts should be soaped or oiled.

Cleaning numnahs

Quilted cotton, linen-covered foam and synthetic sheepskin numnahs should be shaken or brushed after every use and washed by hand or machine when necessary. Some horses have sensitive skin in which case soap flakes or a suitable washing powder should be used. Sheepskin numnahs must be washed by hand in soap flakes, rinsed and have oil applied to the skin side to prevent it hardening.

Cleaning bridles

Hang the bridle up and remove the bit or bits which should be soaked in warm water, hang the reins up and take the rest of the bridle apart, remembering which holes the pieces were done up on. All the leather should be cleaned and soaped as described above and the bit washed, dried and the rings polished. If oiling is necessary this is the time to do it and to check stitching and the condition of the leather where it is folded or bent. The bridle should then be put back together again in the following order (Fig. 6.1):

- The headpiece should be threaded through the browband, ensuring that the throatlash is to the rear.
- The headpiece should be hung on a hook – for a double bridle the bridoon headpiece (sliphead) should be threaded through the near side of the browband, first under the main headpiece and buckled on the off side.
- The noseband headpiece should be threaded through the browband from the off side to buckle on the near side. It should lie under the headpiece.
- The two cheekpieces should now be attached. A double bridle will have two buckles on each side.
- The bit or bits should be attached the right way up and the lip strap if fitted put on. The lip strap should be pushed through the 'D's on the bit from the inner side to the outer side and buckled on the near side.
- All straps should be placed in their runners and keepers and the noseband placed around the bridle and secured by a runner and keeper.

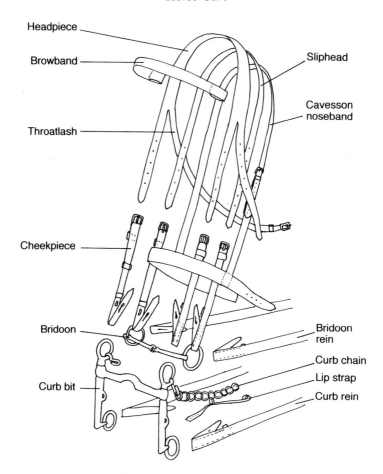

Fig. 6.1 Assembling a double bridle.

● The reins should be replaced; on a double bridle the wider rein attaches to the bridoon while the narrower rein goes on the curb bit.

● The curb chain should be hooked on with the lip strap ring hanging down and the lip strap then fastened through the ring to prevent the chain being lost.

● The bridle can then be 'put up' by passing the throatlash around the bridle in a figure of eight, through the reins and securing by a keeper and runner.

Remember, buckle fastening always goes to the outside while billets (fixed hooks) go on the inside. The rough or flesh side of the leather goes against the horse's skin.

Rugs

Rugs are worn in winter to keep the horse warm and dry and in summer to protect him from flies and to keep him clean and improve the appearance of the coat. Rugs are generally fastened at the front and then secured by a roller or surcingle round the horse's girth; more recently cross-over surcingles and leg straps have become a popular way to secure a rug effectively.

Types of rug
The many different types of rug on the market are enough to confuse any new horse owner. It is important to buy the right rug and one that will last. The clipped horse will need a minimum of a stable rug and one or more blankets, a sweat sheet or cooler and a summer sheet. If turned out during the day in winter the horse will also need a New Zealand rug.

Night or stable rug
The night rug or stable rug is a heavy-duty rug for use on cool summer nights and all day and night in winter. Traditionally they were made of jute or canvas lined with blanket and fastened with a roller. A number of blankets can be worn under the rug to suit the weather conditions; heavy striped woollen blankets, although expensive, are warm, but layers of thinner blankets may be used.

Man-made fibre and quilted rugs are now commonly used; while expensive they are light, warm, easily washed and tend to stay in place better as they come with cross-over surcingles or similar fastenings (Fig. 6.2). There is also less pressure on the horse's back than when using a roller.

Day rug
The day rug is woollen with a contrasting binding and most stables only use them for special occasions. They are fastened at the front and may have a matching surcingle (Fig. 6.3).

Sweat rug or cooler
A sweat rug or cooler is used to cool off and dry horses after exercise.

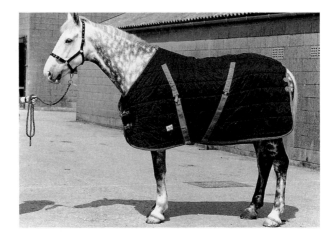

Fig. 6.2 Quilted stable rug with cross-over surcingles.

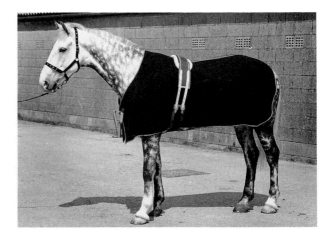

Fig. 6.3 Day rug.

The open mesh type works on the same principle as a string vest, trapping pockets of air to insulate and dry the horse. To work effectively a top rug or sheet must be put over a sweat rug. Coolers are rugs made of material with special properties; the moisture from the horse's body is not soaked up by the rug but taken from the skin/hair through the rug to condense on top of the rug, leaving the horse warm and dry underneath. These make useful travelling rugs.

Summer sheet

The summer sheet is a light-weight rug designed to protect the horse from flies and to keep the dust off the coat in summer. In hot weather it can be used on travelling horses and over the top of a sweat rug (Fig. 6.4). Additionally they can be used as an under-sheet in winter to protect a thin-skinned horse from possible irritation from wool. Washed once a week they help keep the horse's skin and coat clean.

Exercise or quarter sheet

Exercise sheets or quarter sheets can be used under the saddle on cold days or on horses that have been tacked up prior to ridden exercise, for example, race horses in the paddock. The sheet runs from the withers to the top of the dock, reaching down to just below the saddle. It is kept in place by a fillet string and a matching surcingle on the unsaddled horse; if used under the saddle the corners of the sheet are folded back under the saddle flap and girth straps or held in place by loops through which the girth runs.

Hood

A cloth hood can be used in the stable or during exercise to keep the horse warm and thus to prevent the coat on the head and neck growing too rapidly. Stretch or waterproof hoods can be used with a New Zealand rug to keep the horse clean and dry in the field. Hoods can be worn all the time or just when out riding.

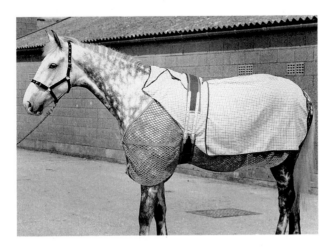

Fig. 6.4 Sweat rug with a summer sheet on top; the front corners of the summer sheet have been folded back and secured with a roller.

New Zealand rug

The New Zealand rug is used to keep outwintered horses and ponies warm and dry and to protect and keep clean the stabled horse which is turned out for a few hours in the day. The rug is made of lined waterproof canvas or synthetic material and is designed to be self-righting so that it stays in position when the horse rolls in the field (Fig. 6.5). The inexpensive types usually have a surcingle stitched to the rug which passes through the sides of the rug and buckles under the horse's belly and leg straps which pass round the hind legs and buckle back to the rug. This design can put pressure on the horse's spine and tends to slip, rubbing the shoulders. More expensive versions may have cross-over surcingles and/or leg straps.

It is imperative that a New Zealand rug fits correctly; it should fit snugly round the neck so that it cannot slip back and press on the withers and rub the shoulders. Some rugs have an adjustable front fastening allowing for the different shapes of horses. The rug should reach to the top of the tail and be of adequate depth. If fitted with a surcingle this should never be knotted to shorten it; take the time to sew it. The leg straps may be made of nylon or leather, which should

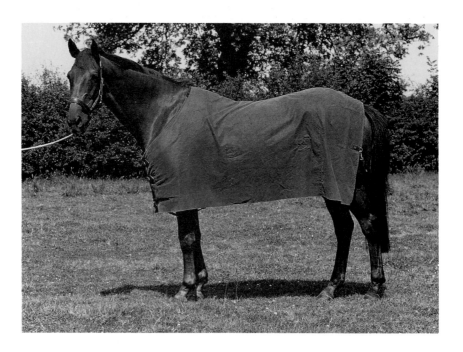

Fig. 6.5 New Zealand rug.

be oiled to keep it soft so that it does not chafe the horse. The strap can be passed round the horse's upper thigh and clipped back to the 'D' on the same side, or crossed to the opposite side; if fastened back to the same side the straps are usually looped through each other. The straps must allow adequate room for movement without dangling by the horse's hocks (Fig. 6.6).

Horses living out in New Zealand rugs should be checked twice a day; a severe rub can develop in a short time if the rug slips. Each horse should have two rugs so that when necessary a dry one can be put on and the other dried. Stitching, leather and buckles must be checked daily for wear, a horse can panic and gallop uncontrollably

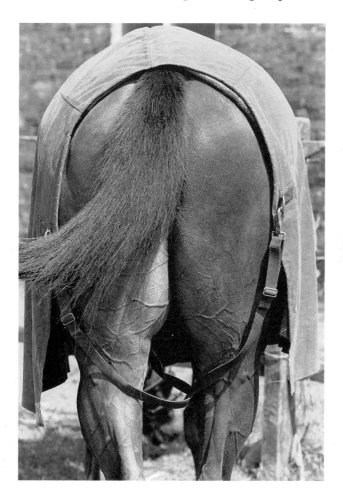

Fig. 6.6 Correctly fitted leg straps.

around the field if the rug slips due to a poor fit or a broken strap. Always catch the horse and get somebody to hold him before trying to adjust a rug in the field; otherwise you may find yourself in a very tricky and potentially dangerous situation.

A young horse can be frightened by a flapping New Zealand rug so initially put it on in the stable to allow the horse to become accustomed to it and then walk and trot him in hand before turning out.

When taking off a New Zealand rug always clip the leg straps back to their 'D's so that they do not hit the horse when you put the rug back on. Clips should always be fastened facing inwards so that they cannot catch on wire fencing.

Keeping rugs in place

Rollers

Rollers are made of leather or webbing and are fastened round the horse's girth to keep rugs in place. Leather rollers are long-lasting but expensive. Webbing or jute rollers are a less expensive alternative, but make sure they are wide enough for the size of horse or they will soon concertina into a narrow band under the horse's girth. A roller has padding either side of the spine, but it may still be advisable to use a thick pad under the roller to minimize pressure on the spine (Figs 6.3 and 6.4).

An anti-cast roller has a metal arch over the withers designed to stop the horse getting cast. Unless this arch is large it is unlikely to work as it merely gets buried in the stable bed (Fig. 6.7). A thick pad is needed under the roller as it tends to concentrate pressure either side

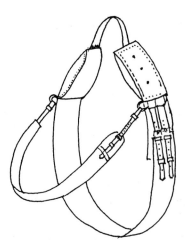

Fig. 6.7 Anti-cast roller with breast girth.

of the horse's withers. There should be buckles on both sides so that it can be undone if the horse does get cast.

Specialist leather rollers can be used for breaking in horses. These have 'D's for side reins, a crupper and a breast girth.

Breast girths

The breast girth is a leather or webbing strap which is fastened to a strap attached to the front 'D's either side of the roller (Fig. 6.7). It is designed to stop the roller sliding back. It should fit closely around the chest just above the point of the horse's shoulder. A similar strap can be used with a saddle, in racing for example.

Surcingles

Surcingles are narrow unpadded straps which hold rugs in place. They are usually stitched into place and care must be taken that pressure is not put on the horse's back.

Cross-over surcingles are stitched at an angle on the off side of the rug, passed under the horse's belly, crossed over and fastened on the near side. These hold the rug in place effectively and with little pressure on the back (Fig. 6.2).

Belly straps

Some quilted rugs have broad bands of matching material which pass from one side of the rug, under the horse's belly and fasten on the other side. Some designs of rug have bands of material which also pass between the front legs in a nappy-type arrangement.

Leg straps

Some night rugs are held in place by leg straps in the same way as a New Zealand rug. Some designs also fasten around the front legs.

Measuring for rugs

Rugs are generally sold with reference to the length of the horse from point of shoulder to point of buttock. For example, a 16hh horse requires a 1.8 m (6 ft) or 6 ft 3 in rug depending on its build. It is worthwhile taking a few more measurements and measuring the rug before buying it. Measure the distance around the horse's neck where the rug should lie; many rugs are far too big around the neck, slip back and sit on the withers. Measure from just in front of the withers to the top of the tail and from the centre of the horse's breastbone to the point of buttock to ensure that the rug will be long enough. A well fitting rug is more comfortable for the horse and lasts longer as it is less likely to get torn.

Putting rugs on (Figs 6.8–6.12)

The horse should be tied up and should stand still while having the rug put on. Always speak to the horse first. If a blanket is worn, collect up the blanket with the left side in the left hand and the right side in the right hand. Fold the blanket in half before throwing it onto the horse's neck. The top half should be drawn back and adjusted so that it is even on both sides and then eased back over the loins to a hand's-breadth from the top of the tail. The front part of the blanket must lie well up the neck and should never be pulled against the lie of the coat; if it is wrong, take it off and start again. It is better to put the blanket on the same way so that soiled areas are always at the quarters.

Unless it is secured the blanket will slip so it is usually turned back over the front of the rug and secured under the roller; both front corners of the blanket should be folded to the top of the withers. The rug should then be either folded and put on like the blanket or gathered up and gently thrown over the neck and withers. The front buckle should be fastened and the rug folded back or eased back over the quarters. The triangle of blanket should then be folded back over the withers, the pad and roller placed on top of the folded blanket and the roller fastened firmly but not tightly.

As long as the horse is placid it is useful to organize the rug and blanket by standing behind the horse to ensure both are even and straight. If attached surcingles are used, they should be checked from the off side so that they are not twisted and then fastened on the near side.

Taking rugs off

Again, no short cuts can be taken; the horse must be tied up and reassured before unfastening the front buckle of the rug. The surcingle or roller should be unfastened, removed and placed over the door, in the manger or, if it is a straw bed, in the corner of the box. Always check to make sure that the rug does not have leg straps or that there is an under-rug which needs unbuckling. The rug and blanket can then be grasped either side of the withers and folded back to the tail. The fold is then held and both rug and blanket are drawn off over the tail. Pulling the rugs off sideways is uncomfortable for the horse and pulls against the coat. The rug and blanket can then be folded and put with the roller.

It is appreciated if the rugs are put ready for the horse's return in such a way that the blanket is folded on top and can be picked up and put straight onto the horse without juggling it and dropping it in the bedding.

In cold weather if there is to be any delay before riding, the rug may be folded back enough to put the saddle on and then folded back over the saddle. If left unattended the horse must be tied up.

Storing rugs

In the spring winter rugs must be mended, cleaned and put away in store; dirty rugs rot and break. Major repairs will require that the rug is sent away to the local saddler to be stitched by machine, but simple repairs such as mending fillet strings or small rips can be repaired by hand at home using a needle and thread. Prompt attention to minor tears will prevent them getting worse and possibly ruining the rug.

Depending on the material, rugs and blankets can either be washed at home or sent away for specialist cleaning. Before washing rugs all leather fittings should be oiled for protection. Some synthetic materials can go into a large domestic washing machine while jute rugs should be soaked in cold water in a trough or dustbin. After soaking, the rug should be scrubbed and thoroughly rinsed before being hung up to dry. Finally, all fittings must be re-oiled. Webbing rollers can be washed providing that the leather is not soaked; it is better to just soak the dirty part of the roller. Leather rollers and leather fittings should be washed clean and treated with a suitable leather dressing. Clothing can be stored in trunks or on shelves in a dry room protected by moth balls. They should be regularly checked for mice which may nest in the rugs or chew them.

Bandages

Bandages are placed around the horse's lower leg to give protection, warmth and support during exercise, travelling or after injury. They must be properly applied as they can cause serious damage if incorrectly put on.

Putting bandages on

Regardless of the type of bandage to be applied there are a few golden rules which will help make the job easier and more efficient:

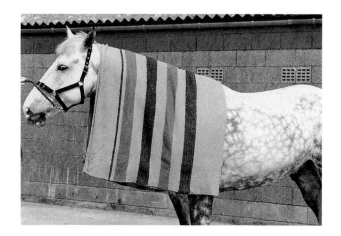

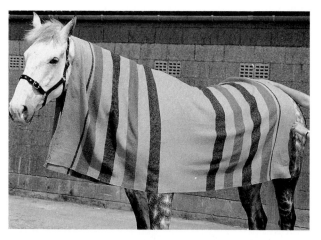

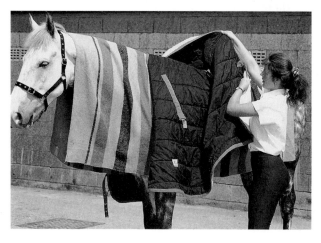

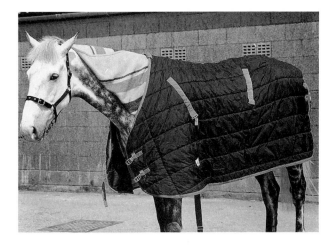

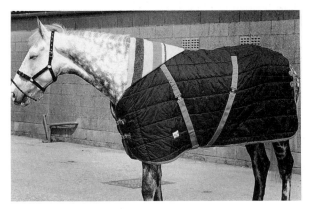

Figs 6.8–6.12 (this page and opposite) Putting on a rug and under-blanket.

- The bandage must have been correctly and firmly rolled up. The tapes must be flat and the bandage rolled towards where the tapes or Velcro are fastened.
- The bandage must not be too tight; there should be room to insert a finger in the top and bottom of a support or exercise bandage.
- The tension throughout the bandage should be even with no wrinkles and the tapes tied no tighter than the bandage itself.
- The bandage is ideally applied from front to back to avoid pulling too much on the tendons at the back of the leg.
- The padding underneath the bandage must always run in the same direction as the bandage and the edge of the padding must not lie

on the tendons or this will cause a pressure point and possible damage.

- The tapes must be tied on the outside of the leg, not on the bone at the front or on the tendons at the back.
- The tapes should be tied neatly in a knot or bow and the ends tucked in to the tape and secured by sewing, insulating tape or pulling one of the folds of the bandage over the tape. It is very important that if insulating tape is used it is not pulled tighter than the rest of the bandage.

Taking bandages off

Untie the tapes and unwind the bandage, moving quickly, passing the unwound bandage from one hand to the other. Once the bandage is off, feel the leg carefully to check all is well. The bandage should then be shaken out, brushed or washed as necessary. Reroll the bandage and store them in twos or fours.

Padding under bandages

Nearly all bandages are applied with some form of padding underneath. The exceptions are Sandown and some thermal bandages which will be discussed later.

- *Gamgee* is cotton wool in gauze cover. Fresh from the packet it is clean and gives good protection, especially wrapped round twice. However, it is easily soiled and expensive. Its life can be prolonged by blanket stitching the edges so that it can be washed and reused. Gamgee is very popular for use over the top of wounds which require bandaging and is frequently an important item of the first-aid kit.
- *Fibagee* is felt-covered foam. It is easy to wash and durable, making it popular for use under exercise and travelling bandages.
- *Leg wraps* are commonly used in the United States. They are thick padded squares which are durable and give good protection, but they are not suitable for use under exercise bandages.
- *Hay or straw* can be used for thatching legs to dry horses and keep them warm.
- *Shaped tendon-protector shells* in a firm synthetic material may be used under exercise bandages.

Fastening bandages

Bandages can be fastened by tapes sewn to the bandage. The tapes should be wide and flat; smoothing them while they are wet will save having to iron them later. A more modern alternative commonly found on stable bandages is Velcro. This must be kept clear of hay and straw or it will not fasten effectively. The two pieces of Velcro must also be long enough to allow sufficient overlap to fasten securely.

Types of bandages

Stable bandages

Stable bandages have several uses and it is important to be able to put them on quickly and correctly. They are used for:

- warmth
- drying off wet legs
- protection, for example, travelling bandages
- support for a sound leg
- keeping a dressing in place.

They may be made of wool or synthetic material and are 10–12 cm (4–5 in) wide and 2–2.5 m (7–8 ft) long. Except for special thermal or Sandown bandages they are always fitted with padding underneath.

If the bandage is being used for keeping a poultice in place or for supporting an injured leg elastic bandages may be used with double gamgee. If the bandage is being used to protect the legs during travelling ensure that the gamgee extends well over the knee and coronet.

The procedure for fitting a stable bandage (Figs 6.13–6.17) is as follows:

- Place the padding round the leg. It should extend about 2 cm ($^3/_4$ in) over the knee and below the coronet.
- If the bandage is long enough start just below the knee or hock.
- If the bandage is short start just above the fetlock so that you are bandaging upwards towards the heart.
- Initially leave a vertical flap of bandage 10 cm (4 in) long. Then the first few horizontal turns secure the bandage.
- Each turn of the bandage should overlap half the width of the bandage.
- Complete the bandage.
- Tie the tapes in a neat bow and tuck the ends in.

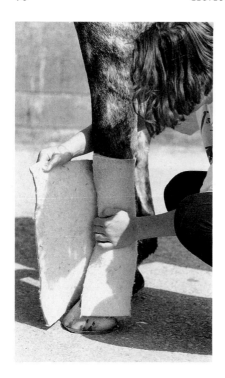
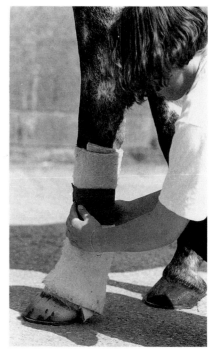
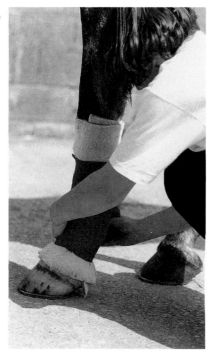
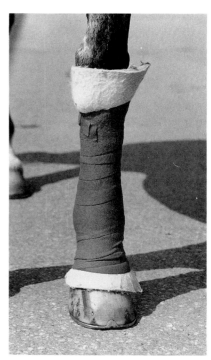

Figs 6.13–6.17 (this page and opposite) Putting on a stable bandage. This bandage is wrinkled and the turns are uneven; it should be reapplied.

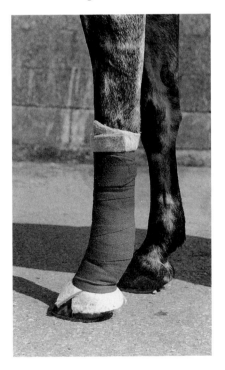

- If the bandage is for support, for example, for a tendon injury, use stretch bandage.

Exercise bandages

Exercise bandages may be fitted on the horse that is working to protect the leg in much the same way as a boot and to support the tendon. It is debatable how much help bandages are in actually preventing tendon strain, but they may help the leg cope with twists and turns.

Exercise bandages have considerable stretch and can be made of elastic, crepe or self-adhesive material. They should be 8–10 cm (3–4 in) wide and about 2 m (6–7 ft) long. It is essential that adequate padding is used under the bandage, for example, gamgee or a tendon-protector shell.

The principles of fitting an exercise bandage (Fig. 6.18) are the same as for fitting any other bandage except:

- They are applied more firmly.
- A longer flap is left initially, for security.

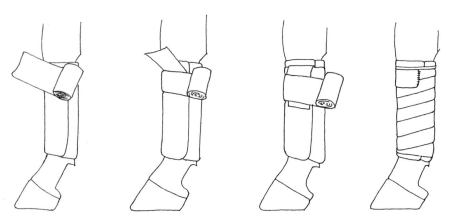

Fig. 6.18 Putting on an exercise bandage.

- They extend from below the knee to the fetlock joint (ergot).
- For competition purposes they are sewn or taped.
- They should not be left on for long periods.
- Overlap two-thirds of the bandage.
- Do not remove from a tired horse until he has recovered.

Tail bandages

Tail bandages are made of stretch elastic or crepe material and are a little narrower and shorter than exercise bandages. They can be used on a pulled tail to improve the horse's appearance in which case the tail hairs are damped with a water brush before the bandage is put on. The bandage should not be left on any longer than four hours; otherwise the pressure may cause the tail hairs to turn white or fall out. The bandage should be applied firmly but not too tightly.

Tail bandages can also be used to protect the tail during short journeys. However, if the horse is travelling for more than four hours a tail guard should be used instead. Bandages can also be used to keep the tail hairs safely tucked away during clipping or when mares are being covered.

To put on a tail bandage (Fig. 6.19):

- If the tail is not plaited, damp it at the top.
- Stand behind the horse and hold up the tail or put the dock over your shoulder.
- Put the bandage under the tail leaving a 10 cm (4 in) flap.
- Secure the end of the bandage and then make one or two turns as high as possible.

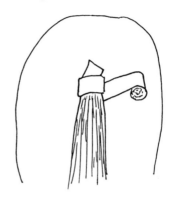

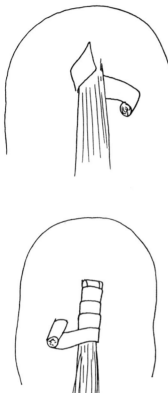

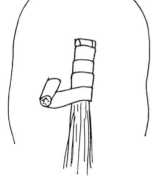

Fig. 6.19 Putting on a tail bandage.

- Bandage down the tail, overlapping about half the bandage at each turn.
- The bandage should reach the end of the dock.
- Wrap the tapes around the tail and tie to the side so that the horse cannot lean on the knot during travelling.

To remove a tail bandage undo the tapes and pull the bandage off with both hands. However, if the tail is plaited the bandage must be carefully unwound.

Boots

Boots are used to protect the horse's lower limbs from injury. Usually the injury is self-inflicted; the horse knocks or treads on himself with another foot. This knock may be due to the horse's conformation, action or shoeing, but could also be caused by fatigue, weakness, immaturity, thoughtless riding, stumbling on landing after a fence ('pecking'), deep going or a change in the ground under foot.

Types of boot

Brushing boots
Brushing boots are designed to protect the inside of the leg below the knee or hock, primarily the fetlock region which can be hit by the other foot at slower paces. The boots should be fitted slightly high to allow for them slipping while the horse is working and should be fastened from the top to the bottom, easing them gently into position. Synthetic boots with Velcro fastenings are very popular as inexpensive exercise boots (Fig. 6.20), while leather boots with buckle fastenings are more suitable for fast work (Fig. 6.21). The boot may be shaped to protect the underside of the fetlock.

Speedicut boots
Speedicut boots protect against high brushing wounds, just below the knee or hock, which can be sustained when the horse is galloping.

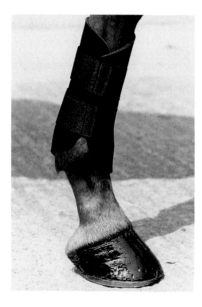

Fig. 6.20 Exercise boot with Velcro fastenings.

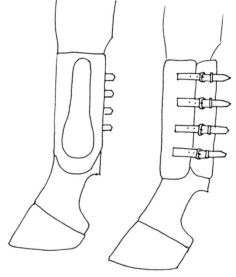

Fig. 6.21 Exercise boots with leather straps.

Over-reach boots
Horses are said to over-reach when a front foot stays on the ground too long and is struck by the inside edge of the hind shoe. This can occur when the horse is jumping and there is an extra effort on take-off or the horse lands in deep going and cannot get its front feet out of the way in time. A low over-reach results in a cut or bruise on the heel while a high over-reach or 'strike' may damage the tendons at the back of the leg.

Low over-reaches may be avoided by using over-reach boots; bell boots are synthetic boots which pull over the hoof or fasten round the pastern to protect the heel and coronet (Fig. 6.22). The boot must not be too long or the horse may tread on it and this type easily turns up in heavy going. A similar boot consisting of petals does not turn up and individual petals can be replaced if they get torn. A tough leather or fabric coronet boot is often used in polo to give added protection to the coronet. Over-reach boots can also be used to protect the horse from tread wounds caused by other horses during travelling or hunting. High over-reaches may be avoided by using brushing boots.

Yorkshire boots
Yorkshire boots are usually used to protect the hind fetlock from low brushing wounds, but their use has been largely replaced by the use of synthetic fetlock boots. They consist of a rectangle of thick material with a tape or Velcro two-thirds of the way down. The boot is wrapped round the leg, tied, eased over the fetlock and the top of the boot turned down (Fig. 6.23).

Rubber rings
A rubber ring with leather or a chain running through it can be fitted either above or below the fetlock (Fig. 6.24). Round the pastern it acts to stop the horse knocking the coronet while above the pastern it prevents brushing wounds. The ring is fastened by a buckle on the strap or chain running through the ring.

Sausage boots
A sausage boot is a large leather-covered padded ring which is fitted round the horse's front pastern to stop the horse bruising or capping his elbow while lying down with his feet tucked under his elbow (Fig. 6.25).

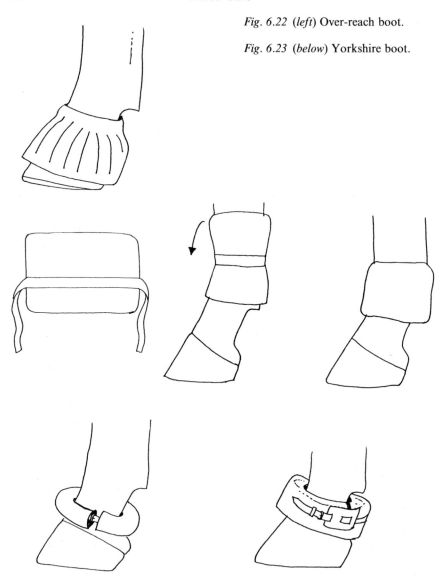

Fig. 6.22 (*left*) Over-reach boot.

Fig. 6.23 (*below*) Yorkshire boot.

Fig. 6.24 Rubber ring.   Fig. 6.25 Sausage boot.

Tendon boots

Tendon boots are similar in design to brushing boots, but they have added padding down the back of the leg to protect the tendons from injury should the horse strike into himself; they are used for fast work or jumping. Open-fronted tendon boots are often used for show jumping; the boot is left open at the front so that the horse is not encouraged to hit fences (Fig. 6.26).

Polo boots

Polo boots are similar to brushing boots, but they are made of heavy felt and extend down over the fetlock and may strap around the pastern (Fig. 6.27). They are designed to protect the fetlock and pastern from bruising by stick or ball.

Travelling boots

Travelling boots are an alternative to travelling bandages and are long padded boots designed to protect the horse from knee/hock to coronet. They are frequently shaped to fit over the joints of the leg (Fig. 6.28). They usually have Velcro fastening and care should be taken when they are first fitted to a horse as the restricted feeling may alarm the horse as he is asked to walk.

Knee boots

Knee boots are designed to protect the horse's knees when exercising on the roads or during travelling when they are used in conjunction with travelling bandages. They may be made of leather, heavy cloth or synthetic material and fasten well above the knee with the buckle on the outside. The top strap usually has a strong elastic insert to allow the boot to be fastened tightly enough to prevent it slipping without damaging the leg (Fig. 6.29). Once the top strap is done up the boot should be eased down to the top of the knee to check that it will not slip over the joint and then the lower strap should be fastened very loosely to allow the knee to flex without interference. This buckle fastens from back to front, which goes against the normal 'rules'.

Skeleton kneecaps or pads are sometimes used for road work and a horse may jump in kneepads which do not have a bottom strap.

Hock boots

Hock boots protect the point of the hock during travelling. There is a top strap with an elastic insert which holds the boot in place and a bottom strap which is fastened more loosely (Fig. 6.30).

Overboots

The overboot is a plastic galosh-type boot designed to fit over the horse's hoof (Fig. 6.31). It can be used on the unshod horse to protect the foot from wear or it can be used as an alternative to a poultice boot

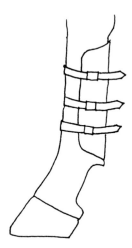

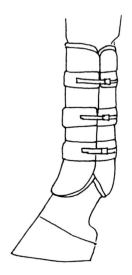

Fig. 6.26 Open-fronted tendon boot.   *Fig. 6.27* Polo boot.

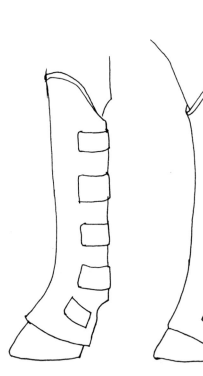

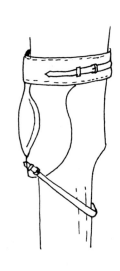

Fig. 6.28 Travelling boots.   *Fig. 6.29* Knee boot.

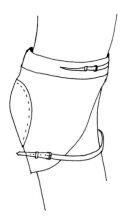

Fig. 6.30 (left) Hock boot.

Fig. 6.31 (bottom left) Overboot.

Fig. 6.32 (bottom right) Poultice boot.

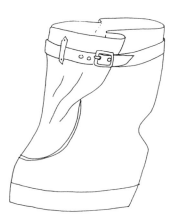

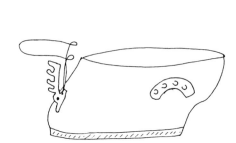

to keep a foot dressing in place. It is also useful for exercising horses during recovery from pus in the foot where the horse may have a tender place on the sole which the boot protects.

Poultice boots
A poultice boot is designed and shaped to accommodate the horse's hoof and lower leg and it is used for keeping foot poultices in place (Fig. 6.32).

Fetlock boots
This boot protects the inside of the fetlock and is sometimes used on the hind legs when show jumping to protect the horse from injury while discouraging him from hitting the fence (Figs 6.33 and 6.34).

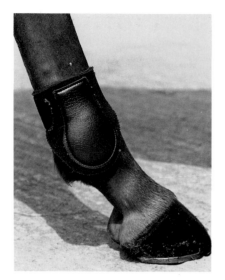 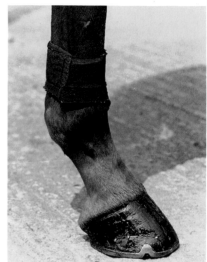

Figs 6.33 and 6.34 Fetlock boot.

Jacuzzi boots

This big rubber boot resembles an equine Wellington boot. When on, it has a hose attached and water circulates inside the boot to cool the horse's lower leg. It is used after strenuous exercise.

7   Preparing Horses for Use

Grooming

Another 'housework ' aspect of horse care is daily attention to the horse's feet and coat. There are several factors that make grooming so important:

- It promotes health by stimulating the blood supply to the horse's skin.
- It improves the horse's appearance, keeping him clean and tidy.
- It helps prevent disease by ensuring thorough daily inspection of the horse's whole body.
- It allows the handler to become familiar with the horse. It is often subtle changes in behaviour that indicate the early signs of illness; the groom should notice these changes first.
- It is a strong contact part of the horse/human relationship.

The grooming kit
The grooming kit consists of several items each of which have a specific use (Fig. 7.1).

The grooming kit must be kept clean and if it is being used on several horses it is likely that the brushes will need a weekly wash in warm soapy water. They should be thoroughly rinsed and left to dry before being returned to the grooming box.

Dandy brush
This brush has coarse, stiff bristles and is used for removing mud and dried sweat from the body and limbs. It should not be used on any horse's head and only with discretion on the body of a thin-skinned horse or clipped horse. The hairs of the tail should not be brushed out with a dandy brush or the tail will become thin. It is very useful for grass-kept horses and is the brush used for the first stage of grooming.

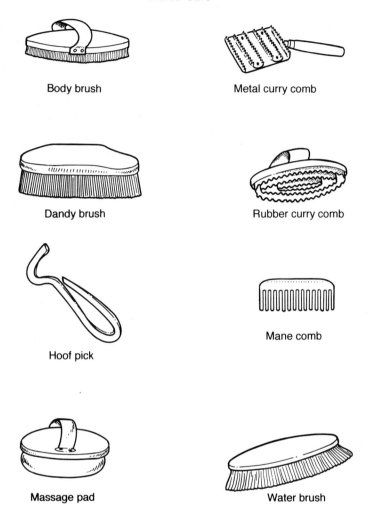

Body brush

Metal curry comb

Dandy brush

Rubber curry comb

Hoof pick

Mane comb

Massage pad

Water brush

Fig. 7.1 Items of the grooming kit.

Body brush
The bristles of the body brush are shorter and softer than the dandy brush. It is used to remove grease and dirt from the coat (Fig. 7.2). The brush is held in the left hand when grooming the near side of the horse and changed into the right hand for the off side. It is used with a circular action to get deep into the coat and loosen the grease, followed by a long stroke to remove the dirt. The body brush is used to clean the horse's head.

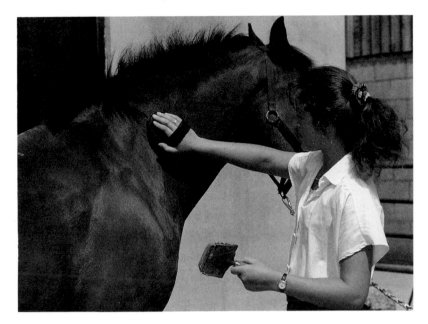

Fig. 7.2 Using the body brush.

Curry comb

The curry comb is held in the other hand and used to clean the body brush; the body brush is swept over the curry comb every four or five strokes. The accumulated dirt is tapped out of the curry comb at regular intervals. The metal curry comb with rows of teeth is only ever used to clean the body brush; using it on the horse's body would cause considerable discomfort. However, the rubber or plastic curry comb can be very useful for removing dirt and hair when the horse is shedding his coat.

Water brush

The water brush has fairly long soft bristles and is used to dampen the mane and tail before plaiting or to encourage the mane to lie flat or before applying a tail bandage. It can also be used to scrub the legs or feet clean.

Sponge

Several sponges will be needed: one for the eyes, nose and lips, one for the dock and sheath (these should be marked so that they are not mixed up), and a large sponge for washing the horse down or removing stable stains. These sponges should be kept for use on the horse and not find their way into the tack cleaning kit!

Wisp

A thorough grooming may include the horse being strapped or wisped. This consists of stimulating the blood flow to the muscles and thus increasing muscle tone, by gently banging the muscles of the neck, shoulders and quarters (Fig. 7.3). It is similar to patting the horse, but a steady rhythm is established using more weight behind the 'bang', and as the horse anticipates the next blow he tenses his muscles. The wisp may be a stuffed leather pad or a traditional wisp made from a length of twisted hay or straw. If the horse is not accustomed to the process, it should be introduced very gently.

Mane comb

A metal or plastic comb is used to comb out the mane, for pulling the mane and tail and for preparing the mane and tail for plaiting.

Stable rubber

This is a linen cloth similar to the type of tea-towel used for drying glasses. It is used slightly damp to wipe over the horse at the end of

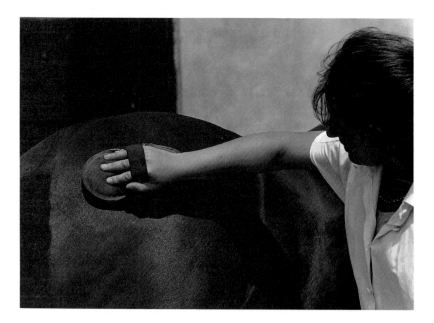

Fig. 7.3 'Strapping' or 'wisping' a horse.

grooming to remove any dust. It can also be used when strapping the horse to wipe the coat flat in between 'bangs' or used instead of the wisp as a folded pad.

Hoof pick
The hoof pick is perhaps the most important item of the grooming kit and yet the one most likely to disappear! It is used to remove mud and stones from the foot and may have a brush on one end to thoroughly clean the underside of the hoof. It should be used from heel to toe, following the contours of the frog (Fig. 7.4).

Sweat scraper
The sweat scraper is used to remove excess sweat or water from the horse's coat after exercise or washing the horse (Fig. 7.5).

The grooming routine
Horses are usually groomed twice a day: a quick brush over in the morning to make them respectable enough to go out on exercise and then a thorough groom in the afternoon or after exercise.

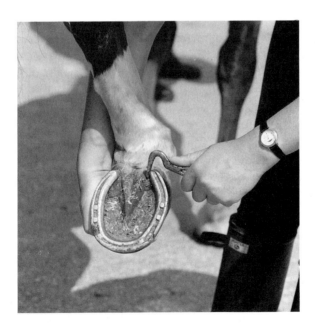

Fig. 7.4 Picking out the foot.

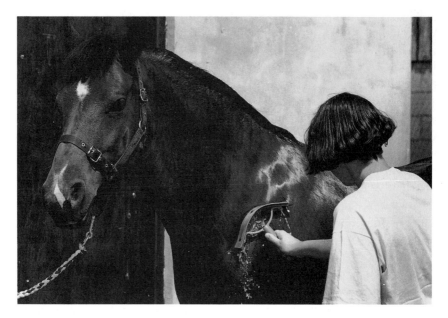

Fig. 7.5 Using a sweat scraper.

Quartering

Quartering is the grooming given first thing in the morning as part of the early morning routine. After the horse has finished his feed and has been given a haynet the horse is tied up and the feet are picked out. The rugs are turned back and any stable stains brushed or sponged off and dried, paying particular attention to the knees, hocks, under the stomach and other areas that may have got dirty when the horse lay down. The rugs are replaced so that the horse does not get cold and the eyes, nose and dock are sponged. Finally the horse's mane is brushed and any bedding removed from the tail. This quick groom makes the horse comfortable and tidy enough to go out on exercise.

Full grooming of the stabled horse

The thorough grooming of a horse is best done after exercise when the horse is warm and the pores of the skin are open. In some competition and hunting yards it is done as part of the afternoon yard routine if all the horses have been exercised in the morning. However, on competition or hunting days it may take the place of quartering in the morning. An efficient groom should be able to complete the task in about 30 minutes, allowing an extra 20 minutes if the horse also needs to be strapped. Obviously grooming will take longer if the horse is very dirty or if the worker is inexperienced.

The horse should first be tied up either in the stable or outside if the weather is suitable, making sure that the yard gate is closed and that the tying up place is safe. In warm weather the horse's rugs can be removed, but in winter a blanket should always be thrown over the part of the horse that is not being groomed.

The horse's feet should be picked out from heel to toe removing all debris and checking for thrush (a fungal infection of the frog) and that the shoes are not loose or worn. The feet can all be picked out from the near side if the horse is accustomed to this practice and the debris may be caught in a skip. If the feet are dirty they should be scrubbed clean over a bucket of water, using a water brush or old dandy brush. Once they are dry, a hoof dressing may be applied.

The next step is to remove any dried mud or sweat from the horse using a rubber curry comb or a cactus cloth for sensitive horses. If the mud or sweat is still damp or if the horse is very sensitive it may be better to sponge the areas clean with warm water and then towel dry the horse.

A thorough grooming includes using the body brush to remove dirt and grease from the horse's skin and coat. Starting on the near side behind the ears, the body brush should be held in the left hand and the curry comb in the right hand. The full strength of the arm should be used to penetrate the coat, working in the direction of hair growth with straight and circular movements. Periodically the body brush should be cleaned on the curry comb and when necessary the curry comb tapped on the floor near the door to get rid of the accumulated dirt. This dirt must be swept up later. When moving round to the off side the brushes should be changed to the other hand and the procedure repeated.

It is a good idea to put the curry comb sharp side down in a safe place when brushing the legs. This allows you to crouch (never kneel or sit) beside the horse's leg and hold the leg steady with the free hand. Holding the tail when brushing a hind leg will help deter the horse from lifting a leg. Remember to stand close to the horse and be firm and positive in your movements.

Once the body and legs have been brushed, the body brush should be used to brush the mane, firmly brushing a few hairs at a time to get right down to the crest. If the mane is tangled a mane comb or plastic curry comb can be used, taking care not to pull out or break the hairs. The mane can be 'laid' by brushing the hairs into place with a damp water brush.

The horse should be untied to brush the head in case he tries to pull back. First brush the front of the face and then undo the headcollar and replace it round the neck and gently brush the rest of the head while steadying the horse with the other hand. Take care to be thorough and not to knock any bony parts. Once completed, replace the headcollar and tie the horse up again.

If the horse needs to be strapped, wisp or bang him for about 20 minutes at this stage in the grooming routine as previously described.

If the weather is cold, once brushing or strapping has been completed the horse can be wiped over with a damp stable rubber and rugged up. The horse should then be untied and a clean sponge used to wipe the eyes, muzzle, mouth and nostrils. The horse can be tied up again and a second sponge used to clean under the dock. Many horses do not like this much so stand to one side, firmly raise the tail and gently but firmly clean the area, rinsing the sponge as necessary.

The tail can now be brushed or fingered through, depending on personal preference and the thickness of the horse's tail. A dandy brush, especially used on a dirty tail, will pull and break the hairs, rapidly thinning the tail. One hand should hold the end of the dock and a few hairs should be separated out at a time removing tangles and bedding. If the horse has a pulled tail the top of the tail can be damped and a tail bandage put on. If not already done the horse's feet should be oiled, the mane laid and the horse finally rugged up, untied and the headcollar removed. Remember to shake out the blankets and rugs before replacing them.

Safety is a prime consideration at all times when grooming. Take care that you do not put yourself in potentially hazardous positions and that jewellery and perfume are not worn; some perfumes make stallions lustful! If you are susceptible to dust a face mask may be worn when grooming to help prevent allergic reactions such as asthma.

Grooming the grass-kept horse
The horse kept at grass needs the grease in the skin and coat to waterproof and protect him from wet weather. This means that he should be cleaned of mud and sweat, but not thoroughly brushed in the same way as a stabled horse.

When brought in from the field the horse should be tied up and the feet picked out and washed, checking the state of the shoes and feet and looking for conditions such as cracked heels. If necessary the feet can be oiled when dry. The mud should be removed from the coat using a dandy brush or plastic curry comb on the body and paying particular attention to the saddle and girth areas which may rub if mud is left behind. The head should be carefully brushed with a body brush, first untying the horse. Sticky sweat marks should be sponged off as should wet muddy legs. The eyes, nose and dock should be sponged and the mane cleaned with a dandy brush or plastic curry comb. The tail can be brushed out with the body brush or fingered through if it is clean. If the tail is dirty it should be washed first.

Cleaning the sheath

Greasy dirt naturally accumulates inside the horse's sheath and some geldings need this area washed regularly to prevent a build up which results in a strong smell and possible risk of infection. The sheath can be washed using warm water and a mild soap with the hands protected by rubber gloves. An assistant may be needed to restrain the horse, either just holding him or picking up a front leg, as some horses may kick out until accustomed to the procedure.

Preparing a horse for competition

Washing the mane (Fig. 7.6)

As always it is important to be organized and the first thing is to gather all the equipment needed: warm water, horse shampoo, a large sponge, towel and sweat scraper. The horse should wear a headcollar, but should not be tied up in case he pulls back. The mane should be wetted with the sponge and a small amount of shampoo worked into the forelock. To prevent the shampoo going in the horse's eyes it may be useful to pull the forelock back between the ears. Gradually work down the mane using the fingers to thoroughly clean the crest. The mane should then be rinsed using the sponge until all the shampoo has been removed. Sweat scrape both sides of the neck and towel dry the ears before brushing out the mane and leaving to dry.

Washing the tail

Collect the washing equipment as before, put on a headcollar and tie the horse up. You may need an assistant for a young or nervous horse. The top of the tail should be soaked using the sponge and the end of the tail immersed in the bucket of water; if the end of the dock goes into the water the horse may drop his hindquarters suddenly. Shampoo should be worked into the tail and rinsed out as before. Excess water can be removed by gently swinging the end of the tail in a circle; stand to one side of the horse when doing this. The tail can then be

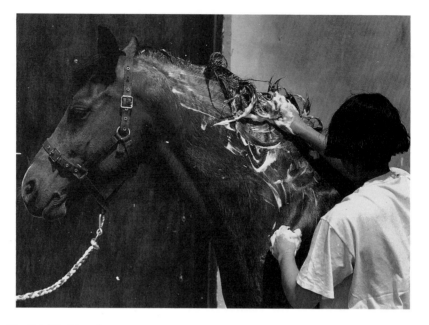

Fig. 7.6 Washing the mane.

brushed or fingered through. Spray preparations to prevent tangling can be applied at this stage.

Bathing the horse
Light-coloured or muddy horses may have to be bathed prior to a competition. To prevent the horse becoming chilled choose a fine day, work quickly and dry the horse off rapidly. If the weather is chilly use warm water; a hose can be used on warm days. Hosing should be introduced carefully as the horse may be alarmed; trickle a gentle stream of water on the horse's front foot, gradually working up the leg until the horse accepts the feel of the water. Wash and dry the head first with the horse untied. Then tie him up to be washed, shampooed and rinsed. Then scrape dry and towel off, paying particular attention to the lower legs and heels. The legs may be bandaged to help them dry and, depending on the weather, the horse lunged or walked with or without rugs to dry off and keep warm.

Washing the legs
Many people wash their horses legs on return from exercise or if they are muddy after being turned out in the field. Care must be taken as

constant washing removes protective grease from the skin resulting in cracked heels and mud fever. If the legs are to be washed use plenty of water and either let the legs 'drip-dry' in a deep clean bed or towel dry and apply stable bandages. The motto is – do it properly or not at all! Barrier cream on the heels and underside of the pastern can help keep the skin soft.

Care of the horse after fast exercise

The hot and sweaty horse needs prompt efficient attention to help his body systems recover effectively. Once the horse has pulled up and the rider has dismounted, the stirrups should be run up and the girths and noseband loosened. If the weather is cold a rug should be thrown over the horse. The horse should be walked until calm and he has stopped blowing. The tack can then be removed and a headcollar put on to restrain the horse while sponging down. In cold weather stand the horse in a sheltered place and use warm water on only the sweaty and muddy areas. In warm weather stand the horse in the shade and use cold water or hose the horse down. Pay particular attention to the bridle and saddle areas. Always avoid wetting the large muscles of the back and hindquarters.

Surplus water should be removed with a sweat scraper and in cold weather the horse can be towelled dry and an appropriate number of rugs and type of rug put on before the horse is walked dry. For example, the horse may wear a sweat sheet covered by a stable rug with the front folded back and secured by a roller. Alternatively, the horse can be 'thatched' – an inside-out stable rug is placed over straw and held with a roller. If the weather is hot the horse may only need a sweat sheet with a cotton sheet over the top.

Pick out the feet, wash them and remove studs if necessary before putting the horse in the stable. Check the horse after 30 minutes by feeling the ears to see if he is warm. If he is cold and the rugs are damp change them for dry ones to help him dry off and keep warm. If the horse is dry, brush him off and put on his normal rugs.

Improving the appearance of a horse

Not content with rearranging the horse's way of life, we also alter the way the horse looks, tidying the mane, tail, feathers and coat to suit

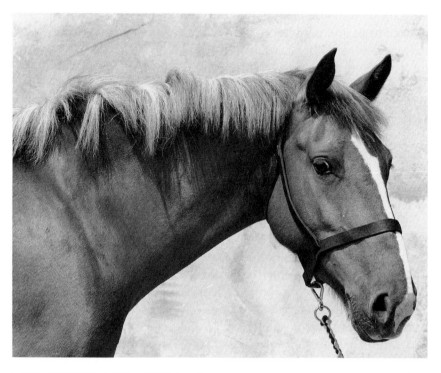

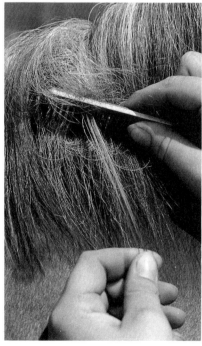

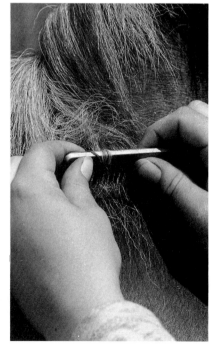

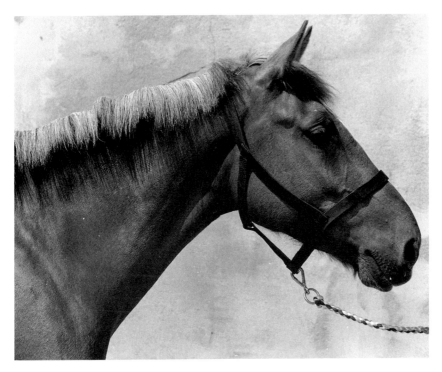

Figs 7.7–7.10 (*this page and opposite*) Pulling the mane. This mane now needs to be put into stable plaits to make it lie evenly.

fashion and the job the horse has to do. Thus, the competition horse and hunter has his mane and tail pulled, feathers and whiskers trimmed and his coat clipped.

Pulling the mane (Figs 7.7–7.10)
The horse's mane is pulled for several reasons:

- to improve appearance
- to thin and shorten the mane
- to make the mane easier to plait
- to encourage the mane to lie flat.

However, Arabs and Mountain and Moorland ponies do not have their manes or tails pulled.

If possible pull the mane after exercise or on a warm day; the pores of the skin will be open making it less painful for the horse when the hairs are pulled out. Some horses object quite strongly to the process and a handler may be necessary to restrain them. Thoroughbred-type horses tend to have fine manes which are easy to pull while part-bred horses can have very thick manes which are tough to pull. Do not wash the mane first as the hairs become too slippery to hold onto and pull effectively. The mane should be pulled so that it lies on the right (off) side of the neck. If it is reluctant to do so, loose stable plaits left in for a day or two followed by regular brushing and damping down will help train the mane.

Method

(1) Comb the mane thoroughly to remove all tangles.
(2) Separate out a few hairs from the underneath of the mane and run the comb up to the roots and remove them with a sharp pull.
(3) Repeat this process until the mane is of the desired thickness and length. Any remaining long hairs from the top of the mane can be shortened by breaking off the ends with the fingers. The forelock is pulled last.
(4) Remove the underneath hairs to ensure that the mane lies flat and grows evenly.

Plaiting the mane (Figs 7.11–7.15)

The horse's mane is plaited to make the horse look smart for competitions, to show the horse off in the show ring or to prospective buyers or to make the mane lie tidily on the correct side.

Equipment

Before starting to plait, the necessary equipment should be collected together. This includes a mane comb, water brush, water and something to stand on. The mane can be secured with thread of a suitable colour, traditionally the preferred method, or with rubber bands. If using thread, a pair of scissors and several needles will also be required. The needle should be of the thick, blunt-ended type used for sewing with wool.

Before starting

It is advisable not to plait the horse in a bedded stable in case a needle is dropped and lost. If this happens, the bedding in the area should be removed, the floor swept and fresh bedding put down. Before starting, it is a good idea to thread several needles with enough thread to do two plaits to save having to rethread the same needle and to place them securely in a piece of thick fabric within easy reach. Plaiting aprons with large front pockets are useful.

Method

(1) Comb out the whole mane and dampen it down using the water brush.

(2) Starting at the poll, divide the mane into as many plaits as required. Tradition used to demand seven or nine plaits, but the modern trend is for many small plaits. A thin neck benefits from larger plaits placed high on the crest while a fat neck can be disguised by smaller tight plaits.

(3) Using the mane comb to keep the remaining mane out of the way, divide the section nearest the poll into three equal bunches and plait down to the end. Pull the hair tightly at the beginning of the plait or the finished plait will look loose and fluffy.

(4) Once the end of the mane is reached, secure by wrapping the thread around it. There are various ways of making the actual plait. One way is to turn the end of the plait under, rolling the plait up towards the neck. Each turn may have to be stitched to keep the plait tight and secure. The plait can then be finished by pushing the needle through the whole plait from underneath and snipping off the thread. This way no thread will be seen. Alternatively, once the ends of the mane are secured the plait can be folded under to bring the end up to the roots of the mane, sewn and then folded again. If the mane is the correct length this will result in a tight ball at the top of the neck. If extra security is needed the needle can be pushed up through the middle of the plait and the thread taken around the plait alternately to the left and right before cutting the thread as close to the plait as possible.

(5) Work down the mane until it is all plaited.

(6) The forelock is done last and can be plaited as the mane or in a similar way to a tail plait (see overleaf). If the horse is restless or head-shy, untie him and get a helper to keep him still.

Removing plaits

Take care when removing plaits; it is all too easy to cut the mane. Use small scissors or an unpicking tool working in the direction of the hair. In time you will be able to use very little thread and remove the plaits

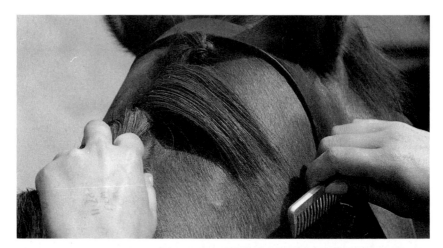

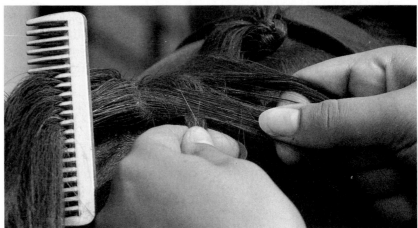

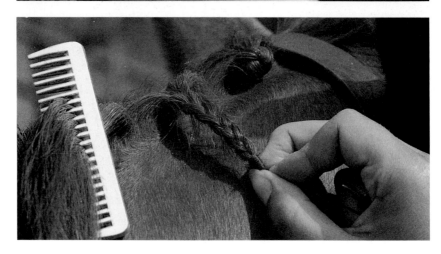

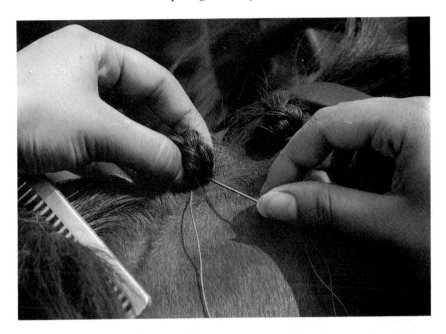

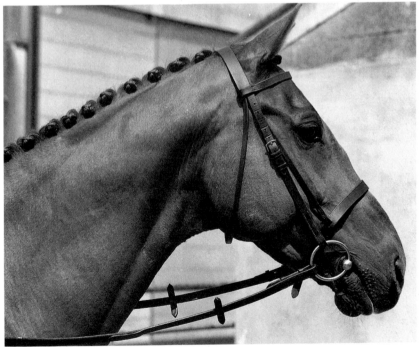

Figs 7.11–7.15 (*this page and opposite*) Plaiting the mane.

with two or three snips. Undo the plait with your fingers and damp down the mane to remove the curl.

Pulling the tail (Figs 7.16 and 7.17)
The horse's tail is pulled for several reasons:

- to improve appearance
- to show off the quarters
- to avoid having to plait the tail.

If possible, pull the tail after exercise or on a warm day; the pores of the skin are then open making it less painful for the horse when the hairs are pulled out. Some horses object violently to the process and a handler may be necessary to restrain them. It is likely that the horse will bleed where each hair is pulled out and it may be better to spread the process out over several days.

Method

(1) Brush the tail thoroughly to remove all tangles and comb out the top.
(2) Separate out a few hairs from the side of the dock, run the comb up to the roots and remove them with a sharp pull.
(3) Repeat this process down each side of the dock until the tail is neat and tidy. Any long hair in the middle of the dock can be shortened or pulled to match the sides.
(4) Side hairs should lie flat and neatly against the dock.

Once the tail has been pulled it can be kept tidy by regular damping and bandaging. As the hairs grow they can be removed on a regular basis – tweaking out a few every day keeps the tail smart without making the horse resentful.

Plaiting the tail (Figs 7.18–7.22)
A full tail may be plaited for competition or hunting. The equipment needed is the same as for mane plaiting.

Method

(1) Wash and brush out the tail.
(2) Separate out a few hairs from either side of the dock and some from the middle of the dock to make the third strand of the plait.

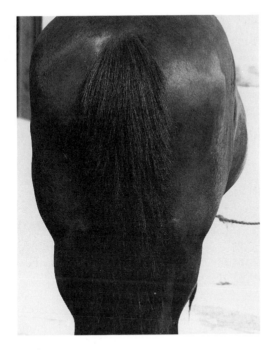

Fig. 7.16 Unpulled tail.

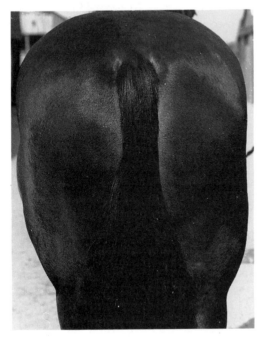

Fig. 7.17 The same tail pulled.

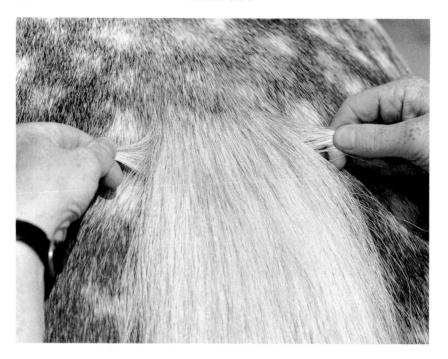

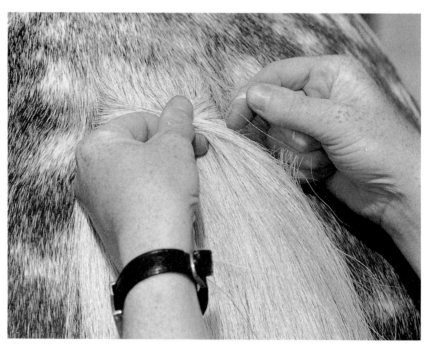

Figs 7.18–7.22 (*this page and opposite*) Plaiting the tail.

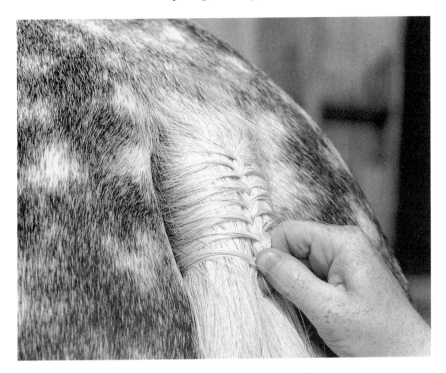

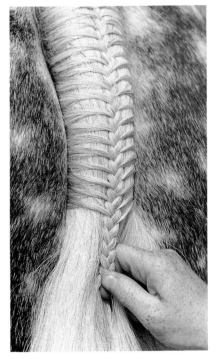

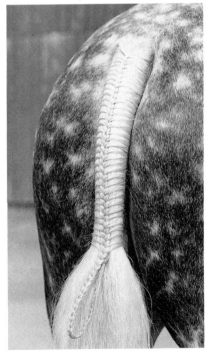

(3)   Plait down the tail incorporating a few hairs from the side of the tail each time. Make sure that the hairs are pulled as tight as possible.

(4)   Continue the plait two-thirds of the way down the dock and then continue plaiting without taking any more hair.

(5)   When the end of the hair is reached, sew it, loop it up underneath and stitch it firmly into place.

A bandage can be put on top of the plait to keep it tidy or for travelling. However, the bandage must not be pulled off but carefully unrolled.

Putting up a tail

Tails may be put up for cross-country, hunting and polo to keep them out of the way. Plait the tail all the way down to the end and secure with a band or thread. Then turn up the plait to just below the dock, double it over and tape or stitch it into place.

Quarter marks

Quarter marks can be used to enhance the horse's appearance; a slightly damp body brush is used to brush the hair in a direction which most flatters the horse. For example, the hair on the quarters can be brushed horizontally towards the tail to make the quarters look longer, while the hair on the barrel can be brushed vertically downwards to make the back look shorter and the girth deeper. Care must be taken that any quarter marks are done really well; poorly done they merely draw attention to that area of the horse.

Clipping

Horses are clipped to remove excess coat; this usually means the thick winter coat that grows in October and lasts until about March.

Reasons for clipping

- To avoid heavy sweating and loss of condition.
- So that the horse can work longer and faster without distress.
- To make the horse easier to clean.
- To dry the horse off quicker thus avoiding chills.
- To improve appearance.

When to clip

The first clip is usually after the horse's winter coat has established in early October. After this the horse may need reclipping as often as every three weeks until Christmas. Horses are not usually clipped after the end of January, once the summer coat has started to grow, as this may spoil the growth of the summer coat. However, performance horses may be clipped in summer to prevent overheating.

Types of clip

Full clip
With a full clip the whole coat is removed. A full clip is used for horses that grow a thick coat or for performance horses, for example show jumpers, in the summer. A triangle is left at the top of the tail to avoid clipping the tail hairs.

Hunter clip (Fig. 7.23)
With a hunter clip all the hair except that on the legs and saddle patch is removed; the hair on the legs gives protection from thorns, mud fever and cracked heels, while the saddle patch is left on to avoid saddle pressure. A hunter clip is used for horses in hard work that are going to sweat heavily.

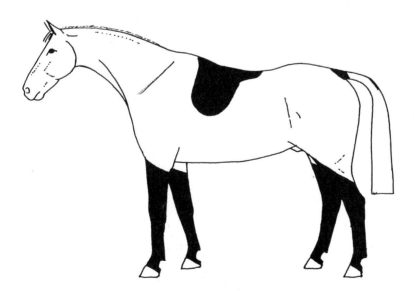

Fig. 7.23 Hunter clip.

Blanket clip (Fig. 7.24)

With a blanket clip hair is removed from the neck and belly leaving a 'blanket' over the back and quarters. A blanket clip is used for horses that feel the cold or are likely to be standing about, for example riding-school horses. It is also used as a first clip for eventers being got fit during the winter months and is useful for young horses that are unlikely to be working too hard.

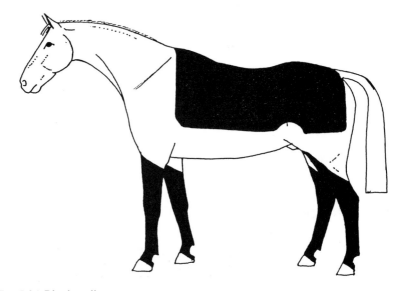

Fig. 7.24 Blanket clip.

Trace clip (Fig. 7.25)

With the trace clip hair is removed from the bottom of the neck, top of the legs and the belly. The head is often left unclipped. A trace clip is useful for horses that are turned out during the day in New Zealand rugs and need some protection from the cold.

Chaser clip (Fig. 7.26)

A chaser clip is a very high trace clip including the head, so called as it is sometimes used for National Hunt horses as it looks smart but still keeps the back warm.

Dealer clip (Fig. 7.27)

With a dealer clip the hair is removed below a line from the stifle, along the bottom of the saddle flap, up the neck and down the side of the face. A dealer clip is a quick clip which makes a horse look

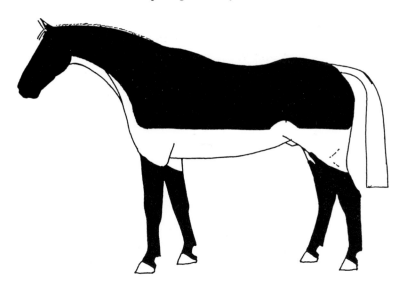

Fig. 7.25 Trace clip.

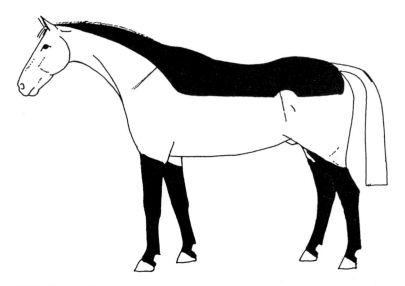

Fig. 7.26 Chaser clip.

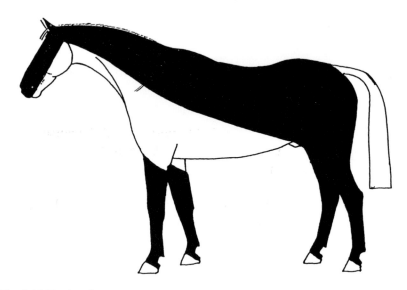

Fig. 7.27 Dealer clip.

presentable, allows it to work and yet still leaves plenty of coat for protection.

Before clipping

Make sure that the clippers have been serviced, are in good working order and have sharp blades. Resharpen blades as soon as they become blunt and keep them in pairs in oiled cloth to prevent rusting. Start with a clean horse – a muddy or greasy coat will soon blunt the blades. Having decided which clip to give the horse, it is a good idea to measure lines with string and mark them with chalk. This will ensure that the lines of the blanket and trace clip are even on both sides of the horse. Finally, bandage the tail and put stable plaits in the mane to keep them out of the way.

Clipping equipment

- Clippers and spare blades
- Oil
- Soft brush
- Paraffin
- Extension lead
- Circuit breaker
- Soft rag

- Rugs and grooming kit
- Assistant
- Twitch
- Dog clippers for head.

The clipping procedure

(1) The handler should wear suitable clothing and the horse should be clipped in a well-lit box. A box with a non-slip rubber floor is ideal although some horses are less frightened if clipped in their own stable.

(2) Assemble the clippers with correct blade tension, oil the clippers and blades and wipe off excess oil. If the horse has not been clipped before allow him to become accustomed to the smell and sound of the clippers before starting to clip.

(3) Start clipping in a safe place on the horse, for example the shoulder. This area is flat and not too sensitive. Move the clippers against the direction of hair growth.

(4) Use long sweeps with firm pressure, moving the skin as necessary in awkward places such as the elbows. An assistant is useful to hold up a front foot so that the skin around the elbow and chest is stretched – this will help avoid nicking the horse.

(5) During clipping keep the air filters clean and oil the blades regularly, checking that they are not hot.

(6) As you remove the hair, keep the horse warm by throwing a rug or blanket over him.

After clipping

Once the clip is completed brush the horse off and wipe over with a damp stable rubber to remove any short hairs left behind. Then rug the horse appropriately. Dismantle, clean and oil the blades and clippers and store them safely, wiping the cables and leads before putting them away. Collect up the clipped hair in a skip and dispose of it.

8   Saddlery

Horses are fitted with saddles, bridles and martingales to enable the rider to sit on the horse securely and to have control. It is important to know about fitting a saddle and bridle and to be able to put them on the horse safely, quickly and efficiently.

Bridles and bits

Bridles can be classified into five families:

- the snaffle
- the double bridle
- the pelham
- the gag
- the bitless bridle.

Under different competition rules, some bits or bridling arrangements may not be allowed, particularly in dressage and Pony Club show jumping.

The leather of the bridle should be of a suitable size and weight for the horse; for example, for showing and dressage light-weight leather may be used while for hunting and eventing heavier leather would be advisable.

Parts of the bridle
The parts of the bridle are basically the same for all types of bridle (Fig. 8.1) and consist of:

- *Headpiece and throatlash.* The throatlash should be fitted to allow a hand's-width between it and the horse's jaw; if too tight it will be uncomfortable when the horse flexes at the poll.

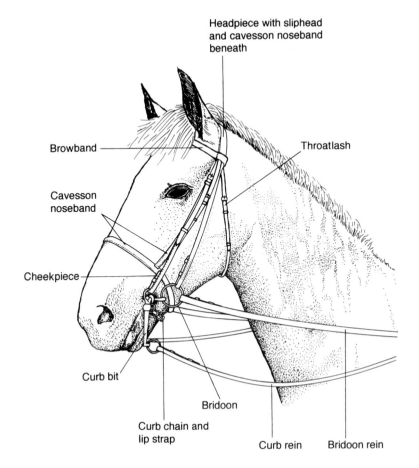

Headpiece with sliphead
and cavesson noseband
beneath

Browband

Throatlash

Cavesson
noseband

Cheekpiece

Curb bit

Bridoon

Curb chain and
lip strap

Curb rein   Bridoon rein

Fig. 8.1 Parts of the bridle.

- *Browband.* This prevents the headpiece slipping back.
- *Cheekpieces.* These attach to the headpiece and hold the bit in place.
- *Noseband.* A simple snaffle bridle has a cavesson noseband which is fitted so that it lies about 2.5 cm (1 in) below the projecting facial crest running down the side of the horse's head. It may be fastened so that two fingers can be inserted between the noseband and the horse's nose or it may be tightened to prevent the horse opening the mouth.
- *Reins.* These attach to the bit and allow the rider to control the horse. Reins may be plain leather, rubber-covered, laced, plaited or made of web with finger slots of leather placed at intervals

(Continental reins). Reins measure from 1.3 m (4 ft 3 in) long for ponies to 1.5 m (5 ft) long for horses and the width varies according to use.

- *Bit.* (This is discussed in more detail below.)
- *Bridoon sliphead.* In the case of a double bridle the bridoon bit has its own support; its off-side cheekpiece attaches to a strap which passes through the browband and becomes the cheekpiece on the near side.
- *Bridoon rein.* This rein attaches to the bridoon bit and is thicker and sometimes slightly shorter than the curb rein.
- *Curb rein.*
- *Curb chain.* The curb chain attaches to the curb bit and may be made of metal, leather or elastic.
- *Lip strap.* The lip strap is a narrow leather strap used to keep the curb chain in place. It prevents the curb chain from being lost.

The action of bits
Bits act on one or more of seven parts of the horse's head (Fig. 8.2):

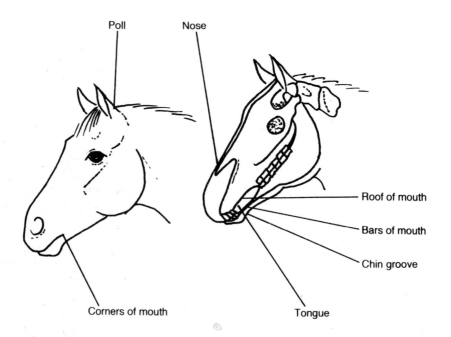

Fig. 8.2 Points of action of a bridle.

- corners of the mouth
- bars of the mouth
- tongue
- poll
- chin groove
- nose
- roof of the mouth.

The action of the bit is affected by:

- the shape of the bit
- the shape of the horse's mouth
- how the horse carries his head and how the rider carries their hands
- martingales, nosebands and other devices.

The snaffle

The snaffle is the most straightforward bit with either a jointed or straight mouthpiece. It acts on the corners of the mouth with an upwards action thus raising the horse's head. The jointed mouthpiece has a more direct squeezing action while the mullen or half-moon mouthpiece has more action on the tongue. However, as the horse learns to accept the bit and flexes at the poll the snaffle acts increasingly on the lower jaw; a drop noseband can accentuate this action.

There are many types of snaffle varying in action and severity (Figs 8.3–8.5). A loose-ring snaffle encourages the horse to mouth the bit and salivate, resulting in a softer contact. A fixed-ring or eggbutt snaffle has a more direct action, but may encourage the horse to lean on the bit and constant pressure will reduce the blood supply to the horse's mouth resulting in poor contact. A horse that is reluctant to take the bit or one that moves the bit too much may go well in a Fulmer snaffle which has cheeks secured to the cheekpieces by short straps called cheek retainers. The French link has a curved spatula in the centre which allows more room for the tongue. Jointed rubber and nylon bits (Fig. 8.4) are useful for young horses which may resent a metal mouthpiece, while mullen mouth snaffles are mild, allowing room for the tongue for horses that cannot cope with a jointed bit.

Generally speaking, a bit with a thick mouthpiece, such as the German snaffle, is mild as it spreads the pressure over a larger area while thin mouthpieces are more severe. Snaffles can also be made more severe by twisting the mouthpiece, as in a twisted snaffle, by

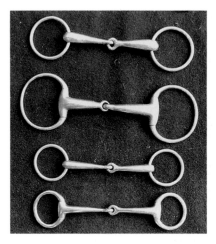

Fig. 8.3 A selection of snaffle bits. From top: jointed German loose ring; jointed German eggbutt; loose ring bridoon; eggbutt bridoon.

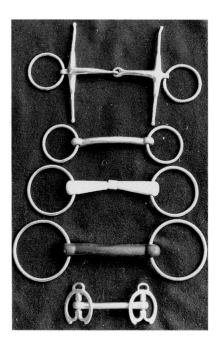

Fig. 8.4 A selection of snaffle bits. From top: Fulmer (or Australian) loose ring; mullen mouth (metal); jointed nathe; rubber mullen mouth; horseshoe cheek mullen mouth stallion show bit.

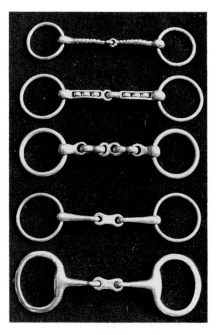

Fig. 8.5 A selection of snaffle bits. From top: wire ring twisted bridoon; Magenis; Waterford; loose ring French link; eggbutt French link.

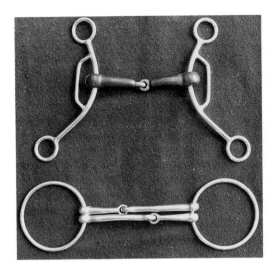

Fig. 8.6 (*top*): American gag; (*bottom*): W-mouth snaffle.

having rollers on the mouthpiece, as in the Cherry roller or the Magenis, or by having extra joints, as in the Waterford or the W-mouth (Fig. 8.6).

Snaffle bits are measured between the rings when laid flat. In the horse's mouth they should fit snugly with about 0.5 cm ($^1/_4$ in) projecting either side of the mouth. If the bit is too narrow it will pinch the horse's lips; if too wide it will slide across the horse's mouth and the joint lying low on the tongue will encourage the horse to try and put his tongue over the bit. An approximate guide to the size of jointed snaffle needed for different horses is:

14.4–15 cm ($5^3/_4$–6 in)   hunter
13.1–13.75 cm ($5^1/_4$–$5^1/_2$ in)   14.2–15 hh and thoroughbreds
11.9–12.5 cm ($4^3/_4$–5 in)   less than 14.2 hh (ponies)

Mullen mouthpieces need to be about 0.75–1.25 cm ($^1/_4$–$^1/_2$ in) narrower to fit correctly.

The double bridle

The double bridle consists of a curb bit used in conjunction with a snaffle or bridoon (Fig. 8.7). This sophisticated arrangement works on many areas of the horse's head giving a fine degree of control. This means that a double bridle should only be used by trained riders on horses that work correctly in a snaffle bridle.

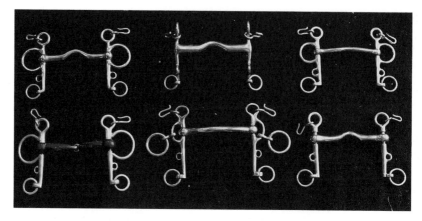

Fig. 8.7 A selection of curb bits (*from top, left to right*): Hartwell pelham (with port); fixed cheek Weymouth; mullen mouth pelham: jointed rubber pelham; Rugby pelham; slide cheek Weymouth.

The bridoon is normally jointed and is thinner and lighter than a snaffle (Fig. 8.3). The curb bit is unjointed with an upward curve called a port which accommodates the tongue so that the bit can work directly on the bars of the mouth. A long-cheeked curb bit is more severe than one with short cheeks as the amount of leverage is much increased. The bridoon acts on the lips and corners of the mouth to raise the horse's head while the curb acts on the bars of the mouth, the poll and the chin groove to flex the poll.

The Weymouth may have fixed cheeks, used in conjunction with an eggbutt bridoon, or a slide mouth, used with a loose-ring bridoon. The curb chain should be adjusted so that it comes into play when the bit is at a 45-degree angle to the mouth.

The pelham

The pelham (Fig. 8.7) is a compromise between the snaffle and the double bridle being a curb bit with one mouthpiece and a top snaffle rein and a bottom curb rein. The action is on the corners of the mouth (snaffle rein), poll and chin groove (curb rein), but the action tends to be indistinct, particularly when roundings are used to allow the use of one rein. (A rounding is a loop of leather running between the two rings of the bit.) The mouthpiece may be straight or jointed, and a vulcanite pelham with its mild mouthpiece and curb action is often useful for horses with good mouths that are strong, for example, over cross-country.

The curb chain should be adjusted so that it lies comfortably in the chin groove and comes into play when the tension on the curb rein increases and pulls the cheeks of the curb bit to an angle of 45 degrees. The curb chain then tightens and has a downward and backward pressure on the lower jaw. Attaching the curb chain through the top rings of the bit allows the curb to have a more direct action and helps stop the curb chain rising up out of the chin groove.

Curb chains are made of a series of linked metal rings which may be single or double (Fig. 8.8). Double linked chains spread the pressure over a larger area and are probably preferable to the more severe single link chains. Curb chains may also be made of elastic or leather. Provided that the leather is kept soft and supple they are less likely to cause rubbing than metal curb chains.

An important member of the pelham group is the Kimblewick (Fig. 8.9) which uses a single rein and is frequently seen on strong ponies. However, horses can learn to lean on this bit and it should not be over-used.

The gag

The gag is a type of snaffle but the rings of the bit have holes in them allowing an extended cheekpiece to pass through and attach to the rein (Fig. 8.10). This means that when the reins are pulled the bit is pulled up in the horse's mouth encouraging the head to be raised. The gag usually has a second rein attached to the bit ring in normal fashion so that the gag rein need only be used when necessary. The gag can be severe and is best used by those who are skilled.

The American gag is useful for strong horses (Fig. 8.6). The rein is attached to the bottom ring and when tightened can exert a very powerful pressure on the poll which acts to lower the head. The leverage is increased by the length of the cheekpiece above the mouthpiece.

The bitless bridle

A bitless bridle acts on the horse's nose and chin groove and is useful for horses with mouth problems (Fig. 8.11). However, it can be severe and should be used with care. The nose and curb pieces must be well padded to avoid rubbing.

Fitting a snaffle bridle

- The browband should fit snugly round the horse's forehead without pinching the base of the ears.

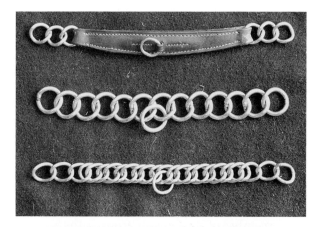

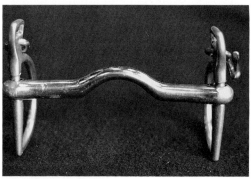

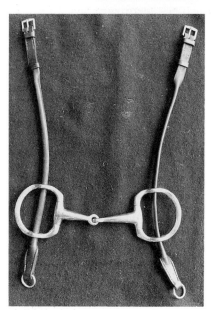

Fig. 8.8 (*top*) A selection of curb chains. From top: leather; single link; double link.

Fig. 8.9 (*middle*) Kimblewick.

Fig. 8.10 (*bottom*) Gag.

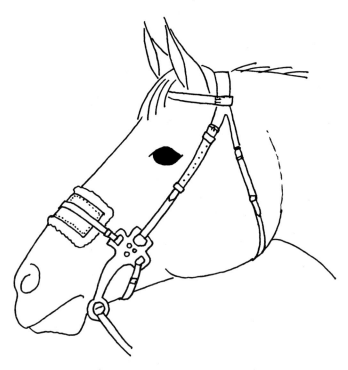

Fig. 8.11 A simple type of bitless bridle.

- The buckles of the cheekpieces onto the headpiece should be an even height on both sides and preferably just above eye level.
- The bit should just wrinkle the corners of the mouth with 0.5 cm ($^1/_4$ in) showing either side – the bit should be pulled straight in the horse's mouth to check its width. The mouth should be opened to check that the bit clears the tushes (the canine teeth found in geldings and stallions lying between the incisors and molars).
- It should be possible to fit a hand between the throatlash and the jaw (Fig. 8.12).
- A cavesson noseband should lie two fingers (2.5 cm (1 in)) below the cheekbone (Fig. 8.13) and allow two fingers between it and the jaw when tightened.

Fitting a double bridle (Fig. 8.14)
A double bridle is fitted as a snaffle bridle except:

- The bridoon has a separate headpiece which buckles on the off side

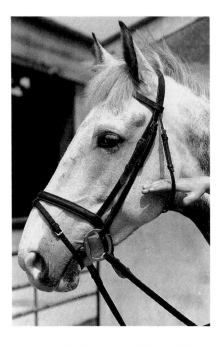
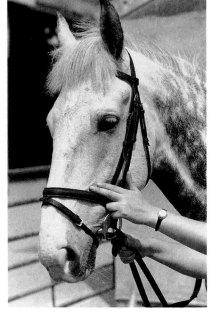

Fig. 8.12 Fitting a snaffle bridle: throatlash.

Fig. 8.13 Fitting a snaffle bridle: noseband.

a little below the buckle of the main headpiece. The bridoon should slightly wrinkle the lips.

- The curb bit is fitted to lie below the bridoon so that it can work separately, but it must not be so low as to interfere with the tushes.
- The curb chain is hooked on to the off side and twisted clockwise so that the lip strap ring hangs down. The flat ring of the curb chain is put on the near-side hook and the selected link is picked up, maintaining the twist to the right and placing it on the hook. If the curb chain is shortened more than three links, equal numbers of links should be taken on each side. The chain must lie flat in the chin groove and remain flat when the curb is used. Double link chains or ones made of leather are most satisfactory.
- The lip strap is buckled on the near side having been passed through the loose ring on the curb chain.

Fitting a pelham

The bit should lie close to the lips without causing them to wrinkle (Fig. 8.15). The curb chain should lie in the chin groove and can be

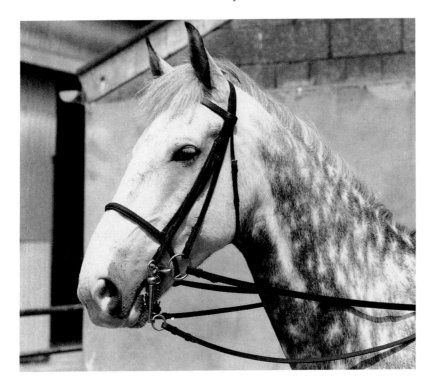

Fig. 8.14 A double bridle correctly fitted.

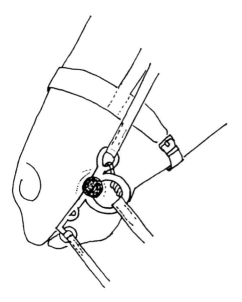

Fig. 8.15 A vulcanite pelham correctly fitted.

placed through the top rings of the bit to prevent chafing. Note that
the curb chain hooks should open outwards away from the horse's
face to avoid injury.

Nosebands

Drop noseband (Fig. 8.16)
This noseband fits around the nose below the bit and is designed to
prevent the horse opening the mouth and thus evading the bit. It
should be fitted so that the front lies on the bony part of the nose; if
too low it will interfere with breathing. The noseband should be
attached to the cheeks to prevent it flopping downwards onto the
horse's nostrils. It must not be fitted too tightly and must allow flexion
and movement of the jaw.

Grakle noseband (Fig. 8.17)
This has two straps which cross over the nose and below the bit in a
figure of eight. It is designed to prevent the horse crossing the jaw and
it is less likely to affect breathing than the drop noseband. It is fitted so
that the headpiece ends just above the facial crest running down the
side of the horse's head. The two straps are stitched together or pass
through a leather pad.

Flash noseband (Fig. 8.18)
This consists of a cavesson plus a strap which passes through a loop on
the front of the noseband and does up under the bit. Again it is less
likely to affect breathing than a drop noseband and it also allows the
use of a standing martingale.

Kineton noseband (Fig. 8.19)
This noseband transfers the bit pressure to the nose and is used on
strong horses. It consists of two metal loops attached to each other by
an adjustable strap. Each loop fits around the bit ring next to the
horse's face so that the centre strap rests on the bony part of the nose.
When the reins are pulled the pull is transferred via the bit to the nose.

Martingales

Competition rules frequently limit the use of martingales and
schooling aids. These rules often apply at the venue as well as during
the competition.

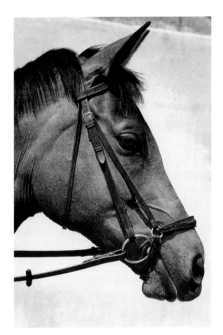

Fig. 8.16 Drop noseband.

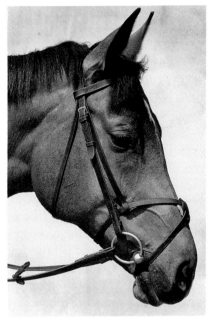

Fig. 8.17 Grakle noseband.

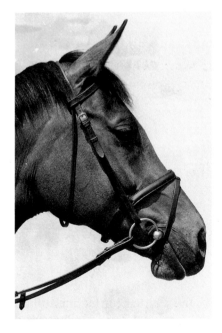

Fig. 8.18 Flash noseband.

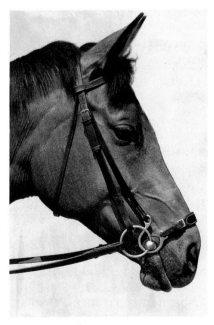

Fig. 8.19 Kineton noseband.

Standing martingale (Fig. 8.20)

A standing martingale has a neck strap through which passes a leather strap with a loop at either end; one end attaches to the girth, the other to a cavesson noseband. The martingale holds downwards on the horse's nose so that the horse does not lift his head beyond the point of control. The martingale should be adjusted so that it does not interfere with the horse when he is carrying his head in an acceptable fashion, nor should it tie him down and prevent him jumping spread fences effectively. When standing in a relaxed position it should be possible to push the martingale up into the horse's gullet.

Running martingale (Fig. 8.21)

A running martingale has the reins passing through the rings of the martingale thus helping to keep the pressure on the bars of the horse's mouth when the head is raised. Correctly fitted the martingale should only come into play when the horse raises his head above a permitted level. The rings of the martingale should nearly be able to reach the withers. A bib martingale has a centre-piece of leather to prevent the horse getting caught up in the branches of the martingale. Rein stops must be fitted on the reins to prevent the martingale rings getting caught on the rein fastening to the bit.

Irish martingale (Fig. 8.22)

An Irish martingale or rings is a short strap with rings like a pair of spectacles, designed to prevent the reins coming over the head in the event of a fall.

Market Harborough martingale (Fig. 8.23)

This has a normal martingale body which splits in two, passes through the bit rings and fastens onto the rein. Its action exerts a strong downward pull on the bit when the horse throws his head up.

Breastplate (Fig. 8.24)

Breastplates are used to stop the saddle slipping back. A hunting breastplate is similar to a martingale with straps running back to fasten to the saddle 'D's'. Care must be taken not to fit them too tightly as they can cut into the horse's chest when jumping. Standing and running martingale attachments can be fitted to the breastplate. An Aintree breastplate is used for racing; this fastens around the chest and is kept in place by a strap over the withers.

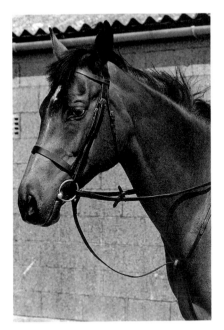

Fig. 8.20 Standing martingale.

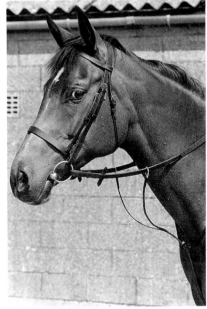

Fig. 8.21 Running martingale.

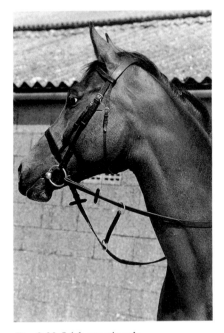

Fig. 8.22 Irish martingale.

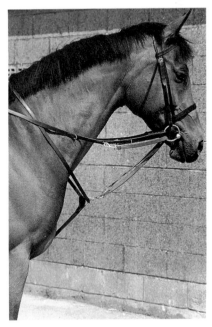

Fig. 8.23 Market Harborough martingale.

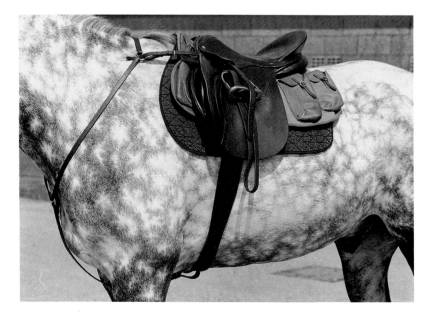

Fig. 8.24 Breastplate. (The saddle is also fitted with a weightcloth.)

Schooling aids

Most schooling aids are designed to teach the horse to lower and stretch the head and neck, thus stretching the muscles of the back and allowing the horse to engage the hindquarters. Schooling aids are common throughout much of Europe and elsewhere in the world. However, if misused they can cause accidents and so must only be employed properly by those trained and skilled in their use.

Draw reins (Fig. 8.25)
Draw reins start at the girth, pass through the front legs, through the bit rings and back to the rider's hands. Each rein passes from the inside to the outside of the bit ring. Draw reins should be used with a normal rein placed above the draw rein. The draw rein may also be fitted so that it runs from the girth straps of the saddle, through the bit rings and back to the rider's hands.

Chambon (Fig. 8.26)
The Chambon runs from the girth, between the horse's front legs to the poll and then down to the bit to put pressure on the poll and induce a lowered head carriage. It is used on the lunge with a mild snaffle bit.

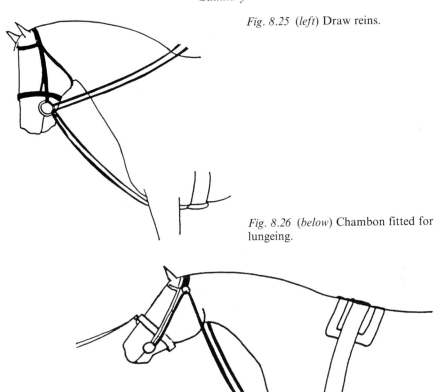

Fig. 8.25 (left) Draw reins.

Fig. 8.26 (below) Chambon fitted for lungeing.

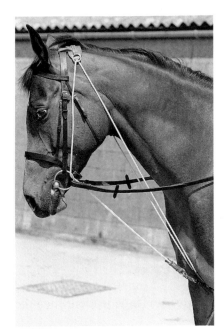

Fig. 8.27 De Gogue.

De Gogue (Fig. 8.27)

The De Gogue is more advanced than the Chambon and can be used for ridden work as well as on the lunge. On the lunge the De Gogue has a strap running from the martingale body to the poll, to the bit and back to the martingale or saddle 'D', forming a triangle. For riding, instead of passing from the bit back to a fixed position, a rein is attached.

Saddles

Parts of the saddle (Fig. 8.28)

Saddle tree

This is the framework of the saddle and its size and shape depends on what the saddle is to be used for. Traditionally it is made of beech-wood but now tends to be made of laminated wood, bonded and moulded, giving a lighter and stronger tree. Racing saddles may have light, fibreglass trees.

The tree may be either rigid or spring: a rigid tree gives strength and solidity; a spring tree (Fig. 8.29) has two flat panels of steel from pommel to cantle and allows the rider more direct communication with the horse underneath them. However, it may tend to concentrate the rider's weight onto a small area and is generally used with a numnah.

Stirrup bars

These are made of forged steel which is riveted to the points of the tree. A hinged safety catch is usually fitted and must never be used in the up position. The bars are placed forward in jumping saddles and further back in dressage saddles.

Seat

Initially webbing is fixed from pommel to cantle and then covered in stretched canvas or linen to form the seat shape. Wool or foam is placed on top as a padding and finally the whole is covered in leather with skirts to cover the stirrup bars.

Saddle flaps

Saddle flaps and girth straps are then added. If the first two straps are fitted to the same webbing piece and the third is independent then the

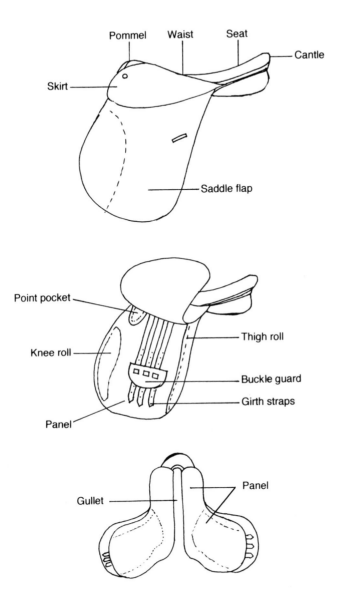

Fig. 8.28 Parts of the saddle.

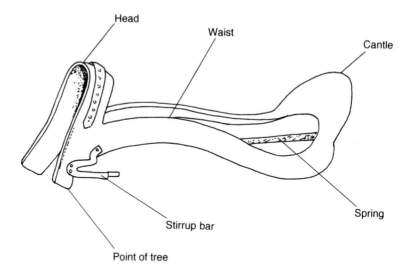

Fig. 8.29 Parts of the spring tree.

girth should be attached to the first and third straps. Dressage saddles may have long girth straps.

Panels
A full panel gives a greater weight-bearing surface and, combined with a wider-waisted saddle, is better for the horse. Thigh and knee rolls are also added to some saddles to help the rider's position. Short or half panels tend to be used on some pony saddles or on show or polo saddles.

Lining
Old saddles may have serge or linen lining, but more commonly saddles are now leather-lined.

Types of saddle

Jumping (Fig. 8.30)
The jumping saddle has forward-cut flaps and knee and thigh rolls to help the rider stay in balance in a forward position. A show-jumping saddle may have a deep seat while a cross-country saddle may have a flatter seat to allow a greater range of movement by the rider.

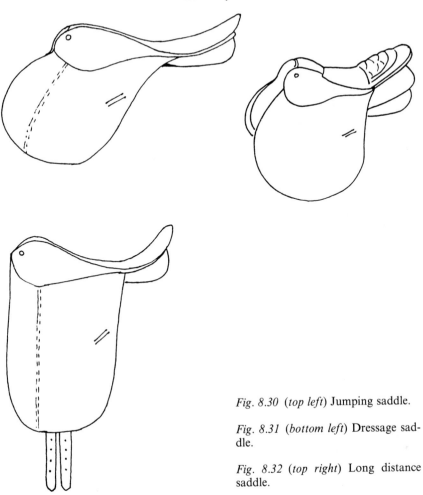

Fig. 8.30 (top left) Jumping saddle.

Fig. 8.31 (bottom left) Dressage sad-dle.

Fig. 8.32 (top right) Long distance saddle.

Dressage (Fig. 8.31)

This saddle helps the rider to achieve a deep seat and a long leg and is straighter cut with a long saddle flap and deep seat. It may have large thigh rolls.

Working hunter

The working hunter saddle is a straight cut show saddle but with knee rolls for showing in working hunter classes.

General purpose

This is more forward cut than a dressage saddle, but still allows the rider to ride with a longer stirrup. It is designed to suit all disciplines, and is also called an event saddle.

Showing
This saddle is designed to show off a horse's shoulder and is only slightly forward cut with a half panel and a relatively flat seat. It is worn without a numnah. Some showing saddles also have a plain flap, no knee roll and a full panel.

Long distance (Fig. 8.32)
This saddle is designed like cavalry and Western saddles to spread the rider's weight over a greater area.

Racing
This is a light-weight saddle with a sloping head and very forward-cut tree. The design varies from the flat race saddle weighing a couple of kilos, or even less, to the more substantial National Hunt saddle.

Polo
This has a reinforced pommel with short panels and long sweat flaps. There are no knee or thigh rolls so that the player can move freely in the saddle.

Accessories

Girths
Leather girths come in three main designs: three-fold, Balding and Atherstone (Fig. 8.33). The shape of the latter two allows the horse's elbow to move while minimizing the risk of rubbing. The three-fold girth has a material insert between the folds which should be kept well oiled. It is fitted so that the fold faces the rear. All three girths may have elastic inserts at the ends of the girth before the buckles to allow the horse's chest to expand while galloping.

The Lonsdale girth is a short girth to fit on dressage saddles with long straps. Care must be taken that the buckles are not fitted where they may chafe the horse.

Synthetic girths are popular, being much cheaper than leather ones. Other girths include string, lampwick and webbing.

All girths must be kept scrupulously clean and regularly checked for wear, particularly where the buckles attach.

Stirrup leathers
These must be of the best quality and regularly checked for safety. The

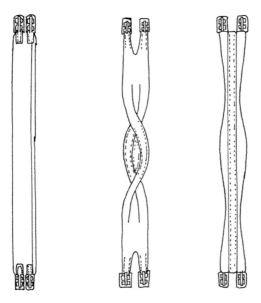

Fig. 8.33 Girths (*from left*): three-fold; Balding; Atherstone.

length and weight of leather will depend on the rider with buffalo or rawhide being the strongest but also the most prone to stretching.

Stirrup irons (Fig. 8.34)
These should be made of stainless steel; nickel is soft and potentially dangerous. The size and weight of the iron must be suitable for the weight of the rider and the discipline, with clearance either side of the foot. Too big an iron is as dangerous as one that is too small. The bent leg (Simplex) safety stirrup is designed for riders who like to have their foot well forward in the iron. Children often use a safety iron which has a thick rubber band replacing the outside of the iron. If the child falls off the rubber band pops off so there is no risk of being dragged. This stirrup is essential with the child's felt pad saddle with 'D's instead of bars. Racing irons are made of light-weight stainless steel or aluminium. Rubber treads are often fitted to the stirrup iron to help the rider keep their foot in the stirrup.

Buying and fitting saddles
The importance of a good fitting saddle for the comfort, well-being and performance of both horse and rider is now recognized, and as a general rule it is wise to buy the best you can afford. For the large

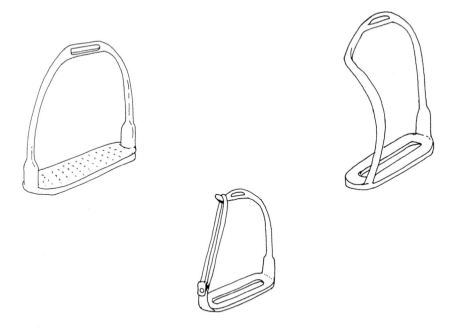

Fig. 8.34 Stirrup irons: *(left)* stirrup with stirrup tread; *(bottom)* Peacock safety stirrup; *(right)* bent leg (Simplex) safety stirrup.

majority of saddle purchasers the services of a competent and experienced saddle fitter should be sought to ensure that a really good fit is obtained.

Saddle fit very much depends on the horse's breeding. For example, a thoroughbred nearly always has a high narrow wither thus requiring a narrow fitting saddle to avoid 'pinching' the withers. Cobs and hunters generally require a fairly straightforward wide fit, but breeds such as Arabs and the New Forest ponies have problems all of their own, to the extent that 'Arab' and 'Forester' saddles have now been developed to cope with their shape.

Remember that the horse's shape changes as it matures and becomes fitter. The shape of the saddle also changes as the padding flattens.

Examining a saddle

The tree should be tested for breakage and damage which may be on one or both sides of the tree. If the front arch is damaged it may widen and come down on the withers. To test the tree place the hands either side of the pommel and try to widen and move the arch or hold the cantle and grip the pommel between the knees. Any movement or cracking sound indicates damage. If the waist is damaged there will be movement when the pommel is placed against the stomach and the cantle pressed up towards the pommel. There is always some give in the seat of a spring tree saddle, but it should spring back into place when released. The cantle should be rigid and any movement would indicate damage. The saddle should be examined for any uneven padding or outline and then placed on a saddle horse to check that it sits evenly.

Once on the horse the width of the gullet should be checked; there must not be any pressure close to the vertebrae. The saddle should sit evenly and level with no tilt towards the cantle or pommel which would unbalance the rider. The panels underneath should be in close contact with the horse's back for the whole length of the saddle. The riders weight should be evenly distributed over the lumbar muscles but not the loins and the saddle must not interfere with movement of the horse's shoulder.

When the rider is on, it should be possible to place three fingers under the pommel, and the horse should be ridden for a few mintues to check that the saddle has not dropped any further. This often happens, especially with a narrow horse. With a new saddle it should be possible to place four fingers under the pommel to allow for the saddle to drop as it is worn in. There must be ample clearance under the cantle and along the gullet and daylight along the gullet when viewed from behind (Fig. 8.35). The saddle must not rock from front to back as this indicates that pressure is not being evenly spread along the length of the saddle. Additionally, the horse should be checked ridden; any undue movement in the saddle will show up then, particularly during rising trot.

Tacking up

(1) Collect the saddle, bridle, martingale and boots (if worn). Check that the throatlash and noseband of the bridle are undone and carry the bridle so that the reins are clear of the ground. Check that the saddle has a girth and numnah attached and carry it over your lower arm with the pommel towards the elbow.

(2) Put the equipment in a safe place outside the stable and catch and

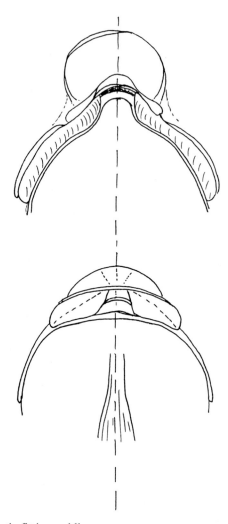

Fig. 8.35 A correctly fitting saddle.

tie up the horse. Remove any rugs, clean the horse as necessary and pick the feet out.

(3) Put on the boots if appropriate.

(4) If a martingale is used fit it before the saddle; untie the horse and pass the neckstrap over his head from the near side. Then tie the horse up again and put on the saddle remembering to put the girth through the loop of the martingale.

(5) Put on the saddle before the bridle in order to allow the horse's back to warm up. With the saddle usually on the left arm,

approach the horse from the near side and pat his back. Then using both hands place the saddle on the withers and slide it back into position. Straighten the numnah, pull it up into the arch of the saddle and attach the girth to the same two straps on both sides, before moving to the off side and fastening the girth, checking that the skin is not wrinkled. Ensure that the stirrup bars are down for safety's sake.

(6) If the weather is cold replace the rug. If the horse is restless fasten the buckles and roller.

(7) Put on the bridle (Figs 8.36–8.38). Carry the bridle and reins over the left arm with the browband nearest the elbow. Hold the bridle up against the horse's head to ensure that the fit is approximately correct. Then standing on the near side behind the horse's eye, reassure the horse, untie him and unfasten the headcollar, maybe placing it round the horse's neck. Pass the reins over the head and, holding the headpiece with the right hand, place the left hand under the bit, guiding it to the horse's mouth. Gently open the mouth by placing the first finger in the gap between the horse's incisors and molars. As the horse opens his mouth , slip the bit in and simultaneously lift the bridle with the right hand. Use both hands to put the bridle over the ears and to tidy the mane and forelock. Adjust the fit as necessary and then fasten the throatlash and noseband and replace the keepers. Put the headcollar back on over the bridle. If it is a double bridle ensure that the bridoon is on top and in front of the Weymouth.

Leaving a saddled horse
The horse should be tied up with the reins made safe; they may be doubled round the horse's neck, twisted and looped through the throatlash or slipped under a stirrup leather.

Untacking

On dismounting, run up the stirrup irons and loosen the girth. Take the reins over the horse's head and lead him into the stable, making sure to turn the horse round and close the stable door. Some stable yards insist that a headcollar is then placed round the horse's neck leaving the rope untied. Then unfasten the noseband and throatlash and release the martingale from the girth. Ease the bridle over the horse's head, steadying his nose and allowing him to drop the bit in his

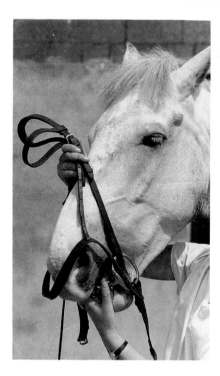

Figs 8.36–8.38
Putting on a bridle.

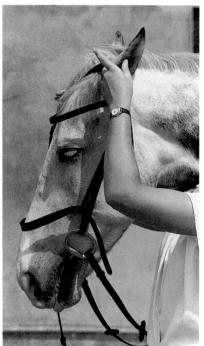

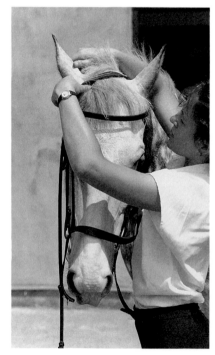

own time. Put the bridle over your left arm, put on the headcollar and tie the horse up. Unfasten the girths and lift the saddle over the horse's shoulder, putting it on your left arm. Turn muddy girths before placing them over the saddle. Then place the saddle on the stable door or on the ground with the pommel towards the ground and the cantle, protected by the girth, against the wall. Lastly remove the boots.

Care of the horse after untacking

After the horse has been untacked pick out the feet and, if necessary, wash off the hooves and heels. Check the legs for heat and swelling. Sponge the saddle and bridle areas to remove sweat marks, at the same time checking for rubs. Then brush the horse and replace the rugs.

9 Feeding and Watering

We have taken horses from the wild and completely changed their lifestyle; instead of roaming freely, eating and browsing plants, herbs and leaves of their choice we have enclosed them in fields and stables. They are dependent on us for all their food and water requirements and it is important to supply these requirements properly if the horse is to remain healthy and do the work we demand.

The 'rules of feeding'

To help us feed the horse several rules of good feeding have evolved. These include:

- Water before feeding.
- Feed little and often.
- Make any changes gradually.
- Feed only good quality, dust-free feed.
- Feed plenty of fibre and succulents.
- Keep feed utensils clean.
- Keep to regular feeding times.
- Feed according to work done, condition and temperament.
- Anticipate feeding requirements, e.g. reduce the amount of feed the day before a rest day.

Behaviour at feeding time

Like all animals horses can become protective at feeding time; this is particularly true in the field where the horse may feel in competition with others and may lash out or bite in an attempt to guard the feed. The feeder must be very aware and safety-conscious when feeding horses both in the stable and in the field.

Horses are individuals and have different feeding habits; some are always greedy, knocking over feed buckets in their enthusiasm while others are more cautious, eating only when the yard is quiet. It is important that the handler is aware of these habits so that any change from normal behaviour can be reported and acted upon immediately; a change in the horse's eating and drinking habits is often the first sign of illness. Once a horse has settled into a feeding routine it is unwise to change the type, time and method of feeding suddenly.

Feeding horses at grass

Hayracks must be of a safe design. The design often used for cattle with a feeding trough underneath can allow seeds to drop into the horse's eyes and may have sharp corners on which a horse can hurt himself (Fig. 9.1). Some round cattle feeders are useful but must be of a type where a horse cannot hit his head or become trapped. The rack must be heavy enough not to be easily pushed over when empty. Racks should be placed in a well-drained spot, away from the fence, with good clearance all round. They should be moved regularly to prevent poaching.

Haynets must be tied securely to a solid fence post or tree (Fig. 9.2) and so that they hang just over the top of the horse's leg when empty, or the horse may get a foot tangled in them. Obviously this is tricky if you are feeding groups of horses as they will be different sizes; in this case, hay is best fed on the floor – wastage is better than an accident. One extra haynet or heap of hay should be put out than there are horses and the nets or heaps should be well spaced so that kicking and bullying is minimized.

Concentrate feeding should be supervised as it is a time when horses

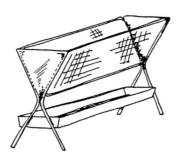

Fig. 9.1 Hayrack and feeder not suitable for horses.

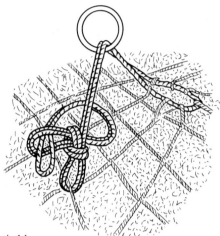

Fig. 9.2 A securely tied haynet.

can be very aggressive and accidents can happen. Always feed all the horses at the same time or take the horse to be fed out of the field and feed it out of sight of the others. There are a variety of buckets and troughs that can be hung over a post-and-rail fence (Fig. 9.3) although these can be knocked off and the contents spilt. Non-spill feeders for feeding from the ground can be purchased including those dropped into a close-fitting tyre. If feeding horses in yards, tethering each horse before feeding ensures safety and that each horse has its share of food.

Worming is covered in detail in *Horse and Stable Management*.

Feeding the stabled horse

Most yards have a feed room containing secure, rodent-proof feed containers with a feed board stating how much and what type of feed

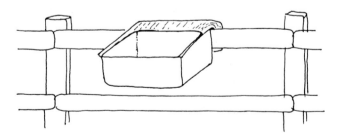

Fig. 9.3 A portable clip-on manger which can be hooked over a fence or the stable door.

each horse should receive in each feed. The quantity of feed may be expressed in 'scoops' in which case the amount of each different feed that a scoop holds should be known – horses should be fed by weight not volume. Some yards use a spring balance and the feed is weighed out for each horse. It is important that everybody understands the feed board and is able to make up feeds.

Horses may be fed in mangers built into the stable, plastic mangers over the door or in buckets on the floor. All utensils used in the preparation of feed, as well as mangers and buckets, must be washed out daily. Hygiene is part of good stable management; it helps in the prevention of disease and ensures that feeds are not tainted which may deter a fussy feeder.

Hay may be fed in haynets, hayracks or loose on the floor. Haynets allow a weighed amount to be fed easily. It is good practice to weight the amount of feed a horse receives – there is less wastage and the hay used can be accounted for. Hayracks are easy to use but can be difficult to empty if the horse does not eat all the hay; this sometimes means that rejected hay builds up, becoming less and less palatable. Feeding from the floor is more natural and allows the horse to sort through the hay, but tends to be wasteful with horses treading hay into the bed. A bale of hay weighs between 20 kg (44 lb) and 25 kg (55 lb) and usually falls into slices when the bale is opened, the slices varying in weight but often about 2 kg (4.4 lb).

If a mouldy and dusty bale is opened it should not be fed, nor should it be soaked in an attempt to make it more palatable. Dusty hay and feed can permanently damage the horse's lungs and handling dusty hay can cause illness in humans.

Simple rationing

The amount of feed a horse needs depends on many factors including:

- size
- condition
- age
- health
- breed
- appetite
- work done
- reproductive status
- environment
- temperament

In practice when a new horse arrives at the yard one has to decide what to put on the feed board immediately; there is no time to get out the

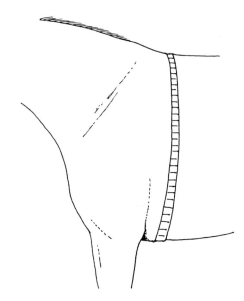

Fig. 9.4 Using a weigh tape. The tape is placed just behind the withers and in front of the girth groove.

calculator! The first thing to do is to decide the size and weight of the horse – large horses eat more than smaller ones. A weigh tape placed around the horse's girth (Fig. 9.4) will give an estimate of the horse's weight and Table 9.1 gives an approximate guide to the relationship of height to weight and the appetites of different weights of horses.

A horse will eat about 2.5 per cent of his bodyweight as dry matter every day. Thus a 500 kg (1100 lb) horse will eat 12.5 kg (28 lb) of feed every day. For example:

Table 9.1 The relationship between height, girth, bodyweight and appetite.

Height (hands)	(cm)	Girth (cm)	(in)	Bodyweight (kg)	(lb)	Appetite (dry matter/day) (kg)	(lb)
11	111.7	135–145	54–58	200–260	440–572	4.5–6	10–13.5
12	121.9	140–150	56–60	230–290	506–638	5–7	11–15.5
13	132.0	150–160	60–64	290–350	638–770	6.5–8	14.5–18
14	142.2	160–170	64–68	350–420	770–924	8–9.5	18–21
15	152.4	170–185	68–74	420–520	924–1144	10–12.5	22.5–28
16	162.5	185–195	74–78	500–600	1100–1320	12–14	27–31.5
17	172.7	195–210	78–84	600–725	1320–1595	13–18	29–40

$$\frac{500 \text{ kg } (1100 \text{ lb}) \times 2.5}{100} = 12.5 \text{ kg } (28 \text{ lb}) \text{ of feed}$$

A rule of thumb that has been used for many years relates the intensity of the horse's work to the ratio of hay to concentrates fed (Table 9.2). The horse in light work will need more hay and less energy feed, while the horse in hard work will need less hay and a greater proportion of high energy feed.

Table 9.2 A guide to the ratio of hay to concentrates to feed according to work done.

Work done	% hay	% concentrates
Resting	100	0
Light	75	25
Medium	60	40
Hard	40	60
Racing	30	70

This means that a 500 kg (1100 lb) horse in medium work has an appetite of 12.5 kg (28 lb) and should be fed 40 per cent concentrates and 60 per cent hay, resulting in a ration of 5 kg (11 lb) of concentrates and 7.5 kg (21 lb) hay.

The next step is to decide what to feed.

Types of feed

Concentrates

Concentrates provide the horse with energy and protein in a less bulky form than hay or grass. Traditionally the horse has been fed cereal grains such as oats, barley and maize; these are high in energy and are suitable for the horse in medium and hard work. However, if fed in excess to horses in light work cereals have a 'heating' effect, making horses too boisterous and difficult to ride. This makes the low energy or 'non-heating' cube or coarse mix ideal for feeding to ponies and horses in light work. Cubes and coarse mixes are compound feeds containing a balanced mixture of energy, fibre, protein, fat, minerals and vitamins. They are formulated to be fed with hay or grass to meet all the nutritional requirements of the horse.

Oats

Oats are the traditional grain for feeding to horses. They can make up all of the concentrate ration of a horse in hard work, but as they are high in phosphorus, limestone flour should be added to the ration. Oats are fed rolled or crimped, but once rolled they begin to lose their nutritional value and should be fed as soon as possible. A good sample of oats consists of plump, golden grains which are free from mould and dust.

Barley

Barley can be fed rolled but is often processed by steaming, micronization or extrusion. Micronization and extrusion are methods of cooking cereals to make them more digestible. Micronization results in large rolled flakes similar to those found in the muesli we eat for breakfast, while extruded barley is reshaped into nuggets by passing it through metal dyes. Barley has a higher energy content than oats and is thus known as a fattening feed. When feeding rolled barley remember that a 'scoop' of barley is heavier and more rich in energy than a scoop of oats.

Maize

Maize is a high energy, low protein and low fibre cereal. It is generally fed steamed and rolled. Traditionally it is only fed as a small proportion of the diet of horses that are not 'good doers' or that lack condition.

Wheatbran

Traditionally bran was fed to bulk out the feed to stop the horse bolting his ration, or as a bran mash. Bran can hold much more than its own weight in water; thus a bran mash has a laxative effect on the gut and is useful if the horse suddenly has to be rested and there is a risk of azoturia. Azoturia is a metabolic disease which may occur when horses in full work and on full rations are rested. When the horse is brought back into work the muscles are said to 'tie-up'. Thus the ration must always be reduced when the horse's work load is reduced. A bran mash is also a palatable vehicle for oral medicines. Bran is deficient in calcium and very high in phosphorus and must be supplemented with limestone flour.

Sugar beet pulp

Sugar beet pulp is the dried remains of sugar beet once the sugar has been extracted. Most horses find it very palatable and it has a fair energy content and a high fibre content. The sugar is digested easily in the small intestine giving 'instant energy', while the fibrous part is fermented in the large intestine, releasing nutrients more slowly. Sugar beet pulp should be soaked before feeding. Shreds are soaked overnight for use the following day and just covered with water. Soak pellets for 12–24 hours using 1 kg (2.2 lb) of pellets in 2 l (3½ pt) of water. Horses can be fed up to 1 kg (2.2 lb) in dry weight of beet pulp per day; this results in about three scoops of wet sugar beet pulp.

Chaff

Chaff is chopped hay and/or straw, usually with added molasses which is added to the feed to stop the horse eating too quickly. It is also useful for ponies on a low concentrate ration. Chaff and horse and pony cubes make a simple ration which can be fed safely by the most inexperienced feeder.

Forage

The design of the horse's digestive system means that he has a high requirement for roughage or fibre – it is his natural diet. The forage part of a horse's diet consists of grass – fresh or conserved as hay, haylage or silage.

All hay contains fungal spores. Soaking hay causes the spores to swell so they are eaten rather than inhaled; inhaling the spores can damage the horse's respiratory system. Evening hay should be soaked first thing in the morning and morning hay should be soaked at evening stables. Alternatively, haylage or silage can be fed. Mouldy or dusty hay should *never* be fed, or soaked in an effort to make it more palatable.

Silage is grass 'pickled in its own juice'. It has a high nutrient value in terms of energy and protein so the concentrate ration will have to be reduced. It can be fed to horses, but once exposed to air it needs eating within two or three days. It is not practical for many yards that lack specialist equipment to move it. Care should be taken to only feed quality silage, as horses have died after contracting botulism from earth-contaminated big bale silage.

Haylage is a compromise between hay and silage; the grass is packed in plastic bales varying in weight from 25 kg (55 lb) to 500 kg (1100 lb). The product is essentially fungal-spore-free and usually highly palatable. It too has a higher nutrient content than hay and may require the concentrate ration to be cut.

Additives and supplements

Additives, for example probiotics and enzymes, are added to an already balanced ration. They may have an indirect effect on the horse's health but they are not fed for their nutritional value.

Supplements are substances added to the horse's diet to balance it by satisfying deficiencies in certain nutrients, most often minerals, vitamins and amino acids.

However, both additives and supplements are not a recipe for success. Horses likely to require a supplement are stabled performance horses, growing youngsters, brood mares in late pregnancy and early lactation, old horses and those receiving poor-quality hay especially in winter. A traditional mixture of corn and hay provides inadequate amounts of calcium for young horses and lactating mares; they will need a supplement.

Supplements vary in complexity; one of the most simple supplements fed to horses is salt (sodium chloride), while at the other end of the scale there are broad-spectrum supplements containing many nutrients. Broad-spectrum supplements are formulated on the basis of the average horse being fed an average ration, making up for likely deficiencies. Some simple supplements cater for specific problems, e.g. biotin for hoof growth.

Guidelines for feeding supplements

- Never mix or overdose supplements.
- Remember that compound feeds are already supplemented; if being fed the amount of cubes recommended by the manufacturers, the horse should not need another supplement.
- Split the supplement between all the feeds.
- If feeding a hot feed like a mash, wait for it to cool down before adding the supplement; otherwise nutrients may be denatured. If feeding a bran mash, be sure to add some limestone flour to compensate for the low calcium level in bran.
- As with any new feed, introduce supplements gradually, taking about a week to build up to the full dose.
- Mix the supplement thoroughly into the feed.

Salt

Whatever diet you are feeding you will need to add salt. The performance horse should have at least 40 g ($1\frac{1}{2}$ oz) per day of common salt added to his feeds, with a salt lick in the manger for insurance. Horses and ponies that are not working so hard could rely on a salt lick either in their manger or out in the field. Grazing horses that eat soil and bark are almost certainly seeking salt.

Calcium and phosphorus
On a grass/hay and cereal diet you will need to add calcium; 25–30 g ($^3/_4$–1 oz) per day of limestone flour is a minimum requirement. Most broad-spectrum supplements contain some calcium and phosphorus but not enough to balance the ration. Requirements will vary depending on the horse's diet, age and reproductive status.

Minerals and vitamins
A stabled horse is likely to require vitamins A, D and E, plus folic acid. A selection of B vitamins may be necessary for performance horses receiving more than 50 per cent of their diet as concentrates. Of all the trace elements, inadequate intakes of copper, selenium, manganese, iodine and zinc are most frequently detected and should be included in a supplement. The form in which the mineral is fed can affect its availability to the horse as well as how it interacts with other nutrients, for instance iron affects the uptake of vitamin E. Unless you are feeding a high quality protein diet, you may have to feed supplements containing lysine and methionine.

Monitoring condition (Fig. 9.5)

Once a ration has been decided upon for a horse and written on the feed board it is vital to monitor that horse's reaction: Does he eat up? Are temperament and performance affected? Is he gaining, losing or maintaining condition? A diet too high in energy may make the horse 'fizzy' and he will grow fatter, while too little energy will result in loss of condition and possibly a lethargic temperament. Some horses are naturally energetic no matter how little they are fed and it must be remembered that training, fitness and discipline will affect temperament. Remember too that a horse must be regularly wormed and have his teeth checked twice a year and rasped if necessary.

Preparation of feeds

Bran mash
Add the required amount of bran to a clean bucket. This is usually about 1.5 kg (3.3 lb), plus a teaspoon of salt and a sprinkling of oats if

Condition score	Back	Pelvis	Comment
4	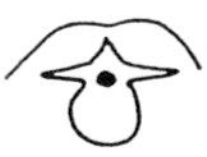	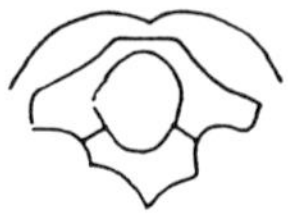	*Obese:* Large masses of fat carried on neck quarters and back. Can only feel ribs on pressure.
3	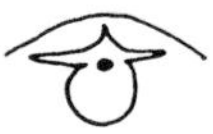	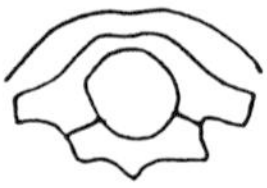	*Getting fat:* Bones becoming more difficult to feel. *Show horses.*
2	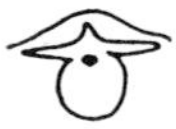	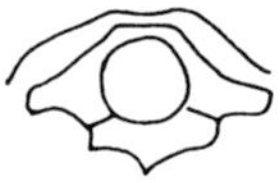	*Approaching normal:* Hip bones and vertebrae of back defined but not prominent. *Hunters & eventers.*
1	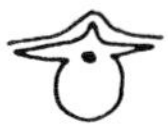	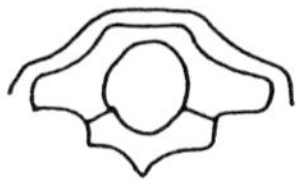	*Thin:* Bones still prominent but a little more muscle definition.
0	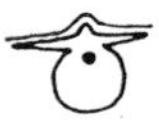	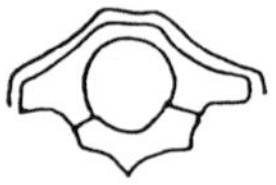	*Starvation:* Croup and hip bones sharp and prominent. Cut-up behind. Rib cage prominent.

Fig. 9.5 Monitoring condition.

the horse needs to be tempted to eat the mash. Pour on as much boiling water as the bran will absorb and stir well. Cover to retain the steam and leave to stand until cool. Before feeding stir in a heaped teaspoon of limestone flour. Correctly made the mash should have a crumbly texture. Molasses or cooked linseed can be added to make the mash more appetizing. A bran mash can be fed to tired horses the night before a rest day or after hard work.

Linseed jelly

Cover linseed with cold water and soak for 24 hours. Allow 0.5 kg (1 lb) linseed per horse. After soaking add more water and bring to the boil. Boil for 1–2 hours until the linseed is soft, taking care that it does not stick and burn. (Soaked linseed that has not been well boiled is poisonous.) Allow the linseed to cool and add the resulting jelly to the horse's feed. To make a linseed mash, add 1 kg (2.2 lb) of bran to soak up the fluid, cover and cool.

Boiled barley
Soak the barley for 12 hours. Then boil gently until the grains are just beginning to split and the water has been absorbed. Boiled barley can be added to every feed if the horse is lacking condition or added to a small feed for a tired horse.

Sugar beet pulp
Sugar beet shreds should be covered with water and soaked for 12 hours. Cubes or pellets should be covered in two-to-three times as much water and soaked for 24 hours. Sugar beet should be freshly made every day as it can ferment, especially in warm weather. Sugar beet pulp is a useful source of both fibre and energy for all horses; it helps the horse put on condition.

The nutrient requirements of elderly horses

Elderly horses need frequent attention to their teeth, as the loss of a tooth or the formation of sharp edges and hooks can cause considerable discomfort, leading to loss of condition. Consequently old horses may need food that is easy to chew; stemmy hay and whole oats would not be suitable as the horse's teeth would not be able to process the food sufficiently to allow adequate digestion.

Nutrition of the sick horse

Providing the horse with a balanced ration plays an important part in the horse's ability to fight illness, and correct nutrition provides one of the body's defence mechanisms. Proper feeding of the sick horse should always be considered as an integral part of the nursing and therapeutic regime.

The task of feeding a sick horse can be difficult and tiresome; the horse's appetite is likely to be depressed, swallowing may be difficult and the function of the gut may be disturbed. Any upset in gut function may lead to dehydration and a disturbance of the electrolyte balance (the ratio of salts in the body), all of which may occur just when the horse's metabolic requirements may be substantially greater. This means that there is often marked weight loss during illness, with a resultant decrease in the horse's defence capacity and prolonged illness and convalescence.

The sick horse's diet must have several special characteristics:

- palatability
- good quality protein
- fibre
- minerals and vitamins.

Palatability

The sick horse must be provided with the most palatable feed possible to encourage eating. Barn-dried hay is ideal if the horse has previously been fed poor quality hay. Maize can be gradually introduced into the diet; it is acceptable and has a high energy content. Molasses, mashes and succulents can all be fed providing that the food is fresh. If swallowing is difficult the feeds should be soft and any carrots cut into very small pieces. If chewing is a problem the horse may need a liquid diet.

Feeding little and often is vital for the sick horse with up to eight feeds a day, including first thing in the morning and last thing at night. Any rejected food should be removed immediately. Soaking or damping the hay may help and will also mean that the horse is taking in water. A smear of vapour rub in the false nostril may mask the smell of medicines in the feed. Plenty of fresh clean water must always be available, and it should be changed frequently. If the horse is using an automatic drinking system, close it off and give the water by bucket so that you can monitor the amount the horse drinks.

Good quality protein

The protein content of the sick horse's diet is more important than the amount of energy the food is providing because the horse is not active, but protein is needed for the repair of body tissue. Good quality grass nuts, milk pellets, stud cubes and soyabean meal are all high in good quality protein; milk pellets have the advantage of being highly palatable. Care must be taken not to overfeed the horse as he recovers.

Fibre

Fibre is important in maintaining normal gut function, but as the fibre content of the diet increases so its digestibility falls and a compromise has to be reached. Molassed sugar beet pulp and bran are useful palatable sources of fibre and can be fed as mashes.

Minerals and vitamins

The sick horse may become severely dehydrated and it is important to supply a suitable source of electrolytes to help restore the fluid balance of the body. A supplement of minerals, vitamins and/or amino acids may be recommended by the vet, depending on the horse's blood profile; an anaemic horse would require iron, folic acid and vitamin B_{12} as well as his normal broad-spectrum supplement. As always calcium and salt are important.

Watering horses

Water makes up 65–75 per cent of an adult horse's bodyweight and 75–80 per cent of a foal's. Water is vital for life; it acts as a fluid medium for digestion and for the movement of food through the gut. It is necessary for growth and milk production and is needed to make good the losses through the lungs, skin, faeces and urine. Restricted water intake will depress the horse's appetite and reduce feed intake, resulting in loss of condition. Under most circumstances the horse should have free access to fresh, clean water at all times. After hard, fast work during which the horse has been denied water, care should be taken to cool the horse before allowing him substantial amounts of water. Excessive consumption of cold water by hot horses can cause colic or laminitis.

The 'rules of watering'

- A constant supply of fresh clean water should always be available.
- If this is not possible, water at least three times a day in winter and six times a day in summer. In this situation always water before feeding.
- Water a hot or tired horse with water which has had the chill taken off it. (This is sometimes confusingly called 'chilled water'.)
- If a bucket of water is left constantly with the horse, swill out the bucket and change the water at least twice a day, topping it up as necessary throughout the day. Standing water becomes unpalatable.
- Horses that have been deprived of water should be given small quantities frequently until their thirst is quenched. They must not be allowed to gorge themselves on water.
- During continuous work, water the horse as often as possible, at

least every two hours. Hunters should be allowed to drink on the way home.

● If horses have a constant supply of fresh clean water there should be no need to deprive the horse of water before racing or fast work. However, the horse's water can be removed from the stable two hours before the race or competition, if thought necessary.

The horse at grass

Access to rivers and streams can be a good way of watering horses at grass provided that the river contains running water with a gravel bottom and a good approach. Shallow water and a sandy bottom may result in small quantities of sand being ingested, collecting in the stomach and eventually causing sand colic.

Ponds tend to be stagnant and are rarely suitable; usually it is best to fence them off and provide alternative watering arrangements.

Filled from a piped water supply, field troughs provide the best method of watering horses at grass. Troughs should be from 1 to 2 m (3 to 6 ft) in length and about 0.5 m (18 in) deep. There must be an outlet at the bottom so that they can be emptied and scrubbed regularly. The trough should be on well drained land, clear of trees so that the ground around the trough does not get poached and the trough does not fill up with leaves. During freezing weather troughs should be checked twice a day and the ice broken if necessary. They must be free from sharp edges or projections, such as a tap, which might injure a horse.

If the trough is tap-filled, the tap should be at ground level and the pipe from the tap to the trough fitted close to the side and edge of the trough. The best method is to have a self-filling ball cock arrangement in an enclosed compartment at one end of the trough. Ideally the trough should be sited along a fence or recessed into it (Fig. 9.6), rather than at right angles to it or in front of it. If not in the fence line the trough should be at least three to four horse's lengths into the field so that there is free access all round and horses cannot be trapped behind it.

The stabled horse

Stabled horses are usually offered water in buckets or automatic drinkers, both of which have advantages and disadvantages.

Buckets

Buckets can be placed on the floor, in the manger, hung in brackets or

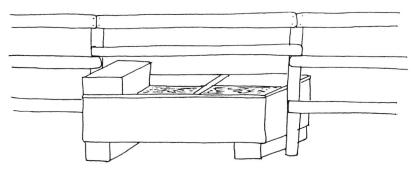

Fig. 9.6 A water trough set into a fence line so that it is accessible from both sides.

suspended from a hook or ring at breast height. They should be placed in a corner away from the manger, hayrack and door, but should still be visible from the door for checking. Providing water in buckets is time-consuming, heavy work and wasteful on water; they must be emptied, swilled out and refilled at least twice a day, and topped up three or four times a day. Horses frequently knock buckets over and may damage themselves by getting a leg caught between the bucket and the metal handle. However, they have three advantages: you can monitor how much the horse is drinking – a change in a horse's drinking habits may be the first sign of illness; buckets are a very simple method of providing water which cannot go wrong; they are cheap – though the cheapest buckets will not last long.

Automatic drinkers
Although expensive to install, automatic drinkers (Fig. 9.7) are an asset in a large yard, saving time and effort. They should be fairly deep so that the horse can take a full drink, they should be cleaned out regularly, sited away from the manger and hayrack, and well-insulated to stop the pipes freezing in winter. Some horses are reluctant to drink from the small noisy automatic drinkers and water intake cannot be

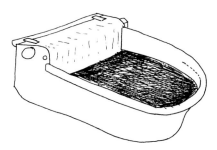

Fig. 9.7 Automatic drinker.

easily monitored. Each drinker should have its own tap so that if it malfunctions, or one needs to monitor the horse's water intake using buckets, it can be switched off.

10   Travelling Horses

Travelling is an important aspect of horse care today. Loading, unloading and travelling are hazardous procedures and it is vital to be well prepared and well practised to minimize the risk of accidents; once a horse has had a bad experience or has travelled badly he can become very reluctant to load and can panic when on the move.

Clothing for travelling

Horses wear rugs and protective clothing during travelling; what they wear depends on several factors including:

- time of year
- weather
- length of journey
- whether the horse is alone or in company
- how well the horse travels
- type of vehicle.

The equipment needed includes the following (see also Fig. 10.1):

- headcollar, rope and poll guard
- sweat rug or thermal travelling rug
- surcingle or roller
- in winter the horse should wear the equivalent of his normal day rugs
- travelling boots or bandages with knee boots, hock boots and coronet boots
- tail bandage and tail guard.

Spare rugs should be available in case the rugs get wet or the horse sweats profusely.

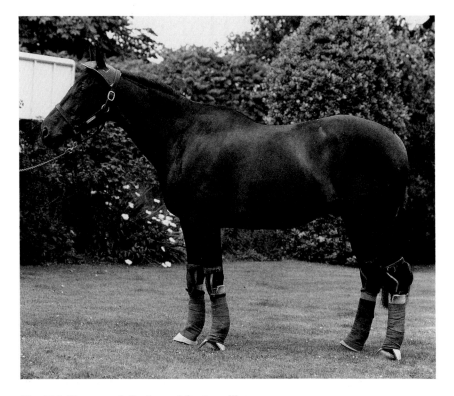

Fig. 10.1 Horse partially dressed for travelling.

Procedure before travelling

Vehicles and trailers must be regularly serviced and checked thoroughly before any journey. Checks should include: the floor and tyres of the trailer including tyre pressure; oil; water; petrol; battery; and lights.

Once the trailer has been hitched up check:

- the coupling hitch and safety chain
- indicators, side lights, brake lights and the internal light
- the jockey wheel and cables are clear of the ground.

It is useful to carry insurance and registration documents as well as your driver's licence. Up-to-date maps and small first-aid kits for both horses and humans are essential. After travelling, the vehicle should be skipped out, the floor swept and left to dry. It is advisable to do this immediately so that the floor is protected from the rotting effect of urine and wet patches. If the weather is suitable the floor may be scrubbed and hosed. Remember to lift the rubber matting regularly so that the floor underneath can be cleaned and left to dry out.

Loading a horse into a vehicle

Loading a fractious horse into a vehicle can be dangerous for both horse and handler and it is wise to think ahead if you do not know how the horse is going to behave. The procedure is as follows:

(1) Position the vehicle alongside a wall so that the horse can only escape one side. Make sure that the gap is very small so that the horse is not tempted to run between the wall and the vehicle.
(2) Avoid slippery surfaces – concrete and tarmac tend to be slippery. If the horse is going to be awkward it may be better to park on grass.
(3) Bed down the floor with straw or shavings so that it looks inviting and is less noisy and slippery.
(4) Swing back and secure the partitions so that the horse is not having to enter a narrow space. It may be better to remove the partitions completely if possible.
(5) Open the jockey door or the front of front-unload trailers so that it is light inside the vehicle and the horse can see a way out.
(6) Make sure the ramp is level and firm so that it does not shift under the horse's weight.
(7) It is very important to have enough experienced help if you suspect that the horse will be difficult; even with well behaved horses it is useful to have an assistant standing by the side of the ramp. The assistant should not stare at the horse as he approaches – nothing stops a horse going forward more quickly (Fig. 10.2).
(8) The handler standing at the horse's shoulder should lead the horse forward and straight up the ramp (Fig. 10.3). It is important not to pull on the horse's head. If he stops, give him a pat, look ahead and walk forward. If he pulls back, do not get into a fight but move back with him until he is happy to move forward.
(9) Once the horse is inside the vehicle, do not duck under the breast bar but stand by his shoulder until the back is secured by

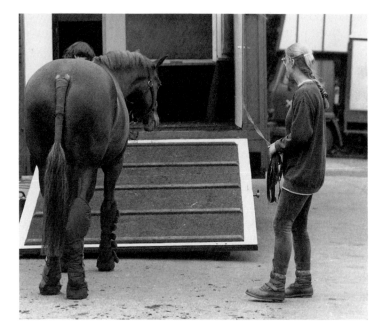

Fig. 10.2 Approaching the horsebox.

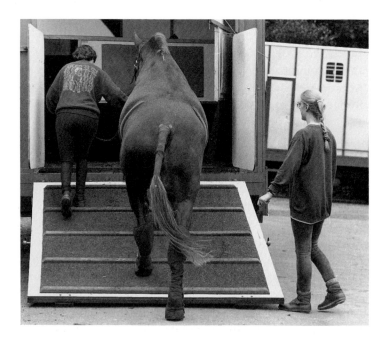

Fig. 10.3 Loading into the horsebox.

the assistant. The assistant should stand to one side when lifting the ramp so that if the horse does rush backwards the ramp will not fall on them.

(10) Once the ramp has been lifted and secured tie the horse to a loop of string so that he cannot swing round but not so tight that he cannot balance himself. The string should be breakable string so that if the horse panics and goes down the string will release him.

If you are on your own then the horse should be loaded in exactly the same way but using a lunge line instead of a lead rope; once the horse is loaded, the lunge line can be threaded through the tie-ring and the tension on the horse's head maintained as the handler backs down the ramp and lifts it. It is important that the horse does not learn that he can rush back down the ramp so never load on your own until the horse is reliable.

Coping with a shy loader

Horses can become difficult to load for many reasons including:

- Reluctance to leave the other horses – position the vehicle out of sight and earshot of other horses.
- Fear of the enclosed space or steep ramp.
- Habit – some horses are 'trained' not to load by inexperienced handlers.
- Memories of a bad journey or forceful loading.

Loading difficult horses should not be undertaken lightly; all handlers should be suitably dressed, including gloves, suitable shoes and a hard hat. The equipment needed includes a lunge whip and two lunge lines, food in a bucket, a snaffle bridle for control or a lunge cavesson.

The horse should be quietly led to the ramp and allowed to look where he is going. If he has a quiet temperament, first one front leg and then the other can be lifted and placed on the ramp, making much of him at each step. If the horse moves back, follow him and start again. This way his confidence can be gradually built up until he is happy to enter the trailer. If a quiet or stubborn horse is not liable to kick, two people can link fingers behind the horse's hindquarters and push him up once his front feet are on the ramp.

Alternatively a lunge line can be buckled to each side of the vehicle, the lines held by two assistants and crossed behind the horse's hindquarters to encourage him forwards. Some horses give in as soon as they realize there is no means of escape while others can lash out or rear against the lunge lines so care must be taken.

Young horses or horses that are reluctant to leave their companions may load more readily if a companion is loaded first. They can gain confidence from the fact that the other horse is not worried by the ramp or the enclosed space. Once the 'problem' horse is loaded, the companion can be unloaded, but take care that the horse does not panic once his friend has gone. Young horses may benefit from the company of an experienced traveller during their first few journeys.

Transporting horses

Many horses become reluctant to load, especially into trailers, after they have experienced a bad journey or forceful loading. Prevention is better than cure:

- Avoid sudden braking, rapid acceleration and fast cornering.
- Use the gears with brakes to decelerate gently into a corner or to a halt.
- Pull away from a standstill or out of a bend steadily.
- Pay attention when travelling over a rough or uneven surface.
- Remember that horses can become frightened if they have previously had a bad experience travelling.
- Overhanging branches and uncut hedges along narrow lanes can be very frightening.
- Trailers towed too fast can start to sway and become so unstable that they jacknife or turn over.
- A speed of 30–35 mph (48–56 km) on normal roads is suitable for most vehicles.

Unloading a horse from a vehicle

The vehicle should be parked in a safe, suitable place with enough room around it. The horse must be untied before the partition, front bar or breeching strap is undone. Many horses can become quite

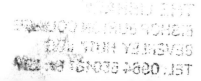

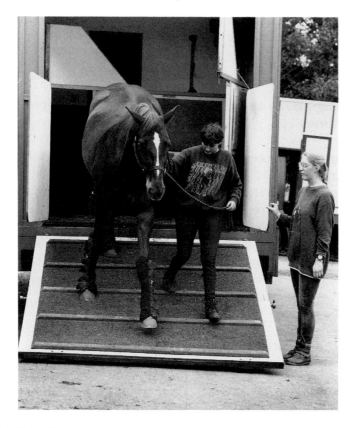

Fig. 10.4 Unloading.

excited in anticipation of being unloaded; they must not be allowed to rush or jump off the ramp (Fig. 10.4).

Care of the horse when travelling

The horse should be kept warm in winter and cool in summer, but remember that the vehicle and the number of horses will influence the temperature and the air available. A single horse in a trailer may get cold, even in summer, while a lorry with three or four horses may become very warm even in winter.

There must be adequate fresh air but no draughts; many lorries are very poorly ventilated. It is better to put an extra rug on the horse and have more air than a warm stuffy environment.

A non-slip floor which makes minimum noise and hence disturbance to the horse will help the horse travel more calmly as will ensuring that horses have adequate space and that the vehicle has suitable suspension.

Travelling mares and foals, inexperienced travellers and stallions

Some horses have special requirements during travelling. A mare and foal will require about twice as much room as normal; the mare should be tied up while the foal travels loose. The partitions may need to be adapted so that the foal cannot pass under them.

Inexperienced or very poor travellers may prefer to travel loose in a large area so that they can find a position that suits them. Studies have shown that travel stress is reduced when horses travel backwards.

Stallions need special partitions to prevent them biting the horse next to them. Alternatively they can be muzzled.

Feeding and watering on journeys

One of the major problems horses experience when travelling long distances is dehydration; it is very important to offer the horse water at frequent intervals. If the horse is sweating it is wise to include some electrolytes. Some horses are more fussy about water than they are about food so take some water from home in a couple of containers so that the taste of unfamiliar water does not put the horse off drinking. If he refuses to drink try adding a little molasses to the water at home so that you can do the same at your destination and disguise the different taste. Fortunately most horses will drink when they are thirsty, no matter what the water tastes like!

The horse will spend a long time standing still during the journey so to avoid swollen legs or any other metabolic upsets the concentrate ration must be reduced. However, in order to avoid loss of condition, allow the horse plenty of good quality hay during the journey so that the gut is kept moving and partially full the whole time; this will reduce the risk of colic. Concentrate feeds should be small, easily digested and given at regular intervals. The horse may be given a bran mash the evening before the journey and only hay or a very small feed, including bran, the morning before setting off.

11   Lungeing

Why lunge?

Lungeing is carried out for many reasons:

- to train the young horse
- to retrain or improve the older horse
- to train the rider
- to exercise the horse
- to warm a horse up prior to ridden work
- for the pleasure of working a horse from the ground.

Some people only lunge mature horses when the roads are too icy to ride on or some other reason prevents their normal riding routine. However, lungeing is a pleasant and useful part of the gymnastic preparation of every equine athlete; the hunter, dressage horse, show jumper, eventer, racehorse, carriage horse and so on will all benefit from lungeing if done well. Similarly it is a pleasing skill in which the lunger gains satisfaction from the quality of the performance. Good lungeing improves a horse's obedience and can be used to build up muscle in the horse as well as developing his rhythm, balance, suppleness and willingness to go forward.

The lungeing equipment

- Bridle – if the horse is being lunged for exercise a snaffle bridle with the noseband and reins removed may be used. If the horse is being warmed up prior to work the horse's normal bridle should be used.
- Lungeing cavesson – this has a padded noseband with three metal rings attached at the front. The lunge rein is fitted to the central ring (Fig. 11.1).

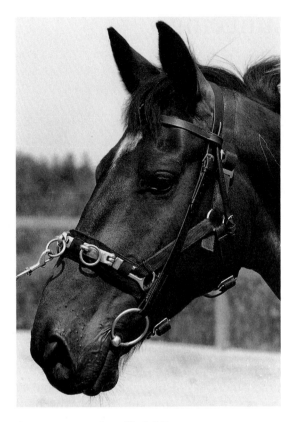

Fig. 11.1 Lungeing cavesson and snaffle bridle.

- Lunge rein, about 10 m (33 ft) long with a large loop at one end and a swivel joint attached to a buckle or clip at the other.
- Side reins.
- Saddle or roller adequately padded with a numnah or pad.
- Breastplate – this may be necessary to stop the roller or saddle slipping backwards.
- Brushing boots.
- Lunge whip.
- Gloves.

Fitting lungeing equipment

The lungeing cavesson has a thick padded noseband which has to be fastened tightly. To achieve this the cavesson noseband of the bridle must either be removed or lie just below the protruding cheekbones. The lungeing cavesson can then be fastened immediately below the noseband of the bridle. Some lunge cavessons fasten below the bit like a drop noseband. The throatlash of the cavesson, if fitted, should not be tight and, as with a bridle, should allow four fingers to be inserted inside the slack.

Further down the cheekpiece, another strap called the cheek or jowl strap should be pulled tight as it helps to stop the cavesson twisting. Care must be taken with a strong horse in case the cavesson pulls round and the cheek strap moves close to the eye. The lunge cavesson should be set over the bridle but the noseband of the cavesson normally goes under the cheekpieces of the bridle to avoid interference with the action of the bit. However, this is not possible with some nylon cavessons. If the bridle has reins attached for riding later, the reins should be twisted under the throat and then passed over the head and secured by passing the throatlash through the loop thus formed.

The lunge line should be clipped or buckled to the centre ring on the front of the lunge cavesson. This ring and the lunge line may be fitted with a swivel; one or other is essential to stop the lunge line twisting as it comes off the coils from the lunger's hands. The lunge line should be soft, strong and long; sharp-edged nylon lines should never be used.

The side reins should be about 2 m (6 ft 6 in) long with a clip at one end and a buckle at the other. The horse should be fitted with a suitable roller with a 'D' ring on each side to which the side reins can be attached. Alternatively, the side reins can be attached to the girth straps on a saddle; this arrangement is normal practice when a horse is being lunged as a warm-up prior to ridden work. The side reins should be passed under the first girth strap in use and secured round the second (Fig. 11.2). The stirrups should be run up the leathers and the loop of the leather passed round the tread of the stirrup and then back under itself towards the rear (Fig. 11.3).

Some people like side reins to have elastic in them and some do not; such discussion calls for a long evening and a drink or two! The side reins should act parallel to the ground, with the horse's head and neck in a posture similar to that when ridden, i.e. the side reins must not be set too low or allowed to slip downwards. The side reins should not be fastened to the bit rings when the horse is first tacked up; they should be clipped to the roller or saddle (Fig. 11.3). This arrangement should be adopted until the horse has relaxed on the lunge and again at the end of the lunge work.

For lungeing, the horse must wear brushing boots on all four legs;

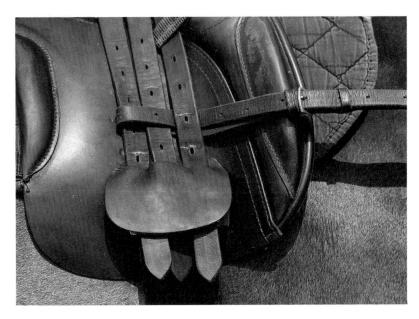

Fig. 11.2 Side rein attached to the girth straps.

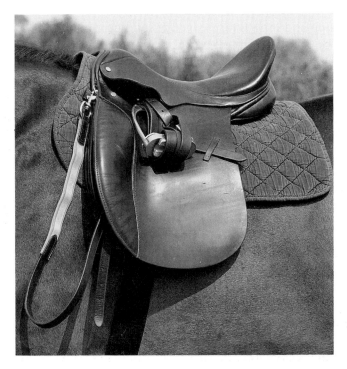

Fig. 11.3 Stirrup leathers secured and side reins clipped up out of the way.

even with sympathetic and disciplined lungeing on a large circle the horse may knock himself, so protection is essential (Fig. 11.4).

Lungers must wear stout footwear in case their toes are trodden on. The footwear should also have a good heel as a smooth under-surface gives poor grip. Properly fitting gloves are essential when lungeing to protect the hands and enhance grip. Those breaking horses on the lunge must wear a hat for obvious reasons; for all others a hat is a matter of preference or exam board protocol (Fig. 11.5). Spurs are best not worn when lungeing.

The aids

The main aid to control when lungeing is the voice. Instead of the horse being between the leg and the hand he is between the lunge whip and the rein; the lunge rein is used to keep a light consistent contact with the horse and if the horse becomes strong the tension on the rein is relaxed and retaken consecutively until the horse stops resisting. The horse should be accustomed to the whip.

Lungeing a horse for exercise

The horse is led to the lunge area with the side reins clipped back to the roller. There are two schools of thought about sending the horse forward from the halt. One method is as follows: the horse is stood on the circle facing for instance to the left. The lunger has the lunge line leading from their left hand to the horse. The spare coils of lunge line may be held in the left hand or, if preferred, in the right hand. This latter style is better for a frisky horse. The lunge whip is tucked under the left elbow, pointing to the rear. The horse should stand still as the lunger takes a few steps back towards the centre of the circle. Not all horses will stand still but such discipline and good practice should be instilled in every horse; it is a matter of patient, calm insistence and consistency.

When well clear of the horse the lunge whip can be brought quietly round behind the lunger's back into the right hand to point a metre (yard) or two to the rear of the horse and towards the ground. The command is 'walk on' but it may be prefixed with either 'and' or the name of the horse; either prefix warns the horse that, whatever else the lunger may have been saying, they are now about to issue a command.

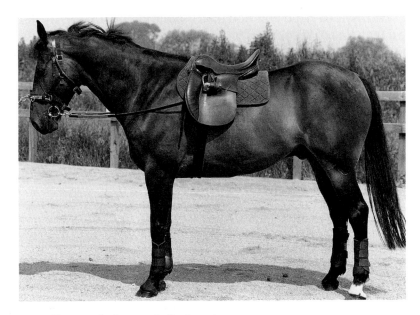

Fig. 11.4 Horse tacked up ready for lungeing.

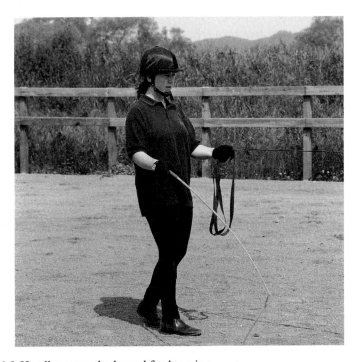

Fig. 11.5 Handler correctly dressed for lungeing.

The 'and walk on' is enforced by raising the whip to buttock height with a little shake that curls out the thong of the whip so it can be seen by the horse. As the walk proceeds the lunger moves on an inner circle, but by gradually letting out the lunge line makes spiral progress to the centre of the circle. This method establishes the horse on the outer track from the outset.

The second and more common method of sending a horse forward in walk is for the lunger to step just clear of the horse before sending him forward using the whip quietly to encourage the horse to go forwards and outwards. Thus the horse spirals outwards. The thinking behind this method is twofold: firstly, it encourages the horse to go away from the lunger rather than the lunger drawing back towards the centre of the circle; secondly, it does not require the horse to be obedient enough to stand still on the circle – many horses will turn in because they have not been taught good behaviour in this respect. Thus this method copes with strange horses and those lunged by many different people, as at a riding establishment. With this method of sending the horse out particular vigilance is required with a fresh or cheeky horse which might plunge forwards and kick out at the lunger.

The walk should be purposeful, long and unhurried with the hind feet overtracking the print left by the front feet. A walk of this quality may not be achieved in the first few minutes, particularly if the horse has just come from the stable.

Control of the horse is subtle and requires both concentration and anticipation. Lungeing is a great skill and, like riding, there is great pleasure in doing it well. If the lunger stands in the centre of the circle they are in a neutral position with the horse balanced between the whip pointing towards him and the taut lunge line; that is to say, equally between the lunger's two hands (Fig. 11.6). If the horse is on the left rein and the lunger wishes to increase the pace, the lunger takes one step to the right. They are now slightly behind the horse and raising the lunge whip a little and clicking the tongue can send the horse forward more purposefully. On the other hand, if the horse is rather too forward, the lunger steps a pace to the left and lowers the whip point towards the ground. Now they are slightly ahead of the horse and with a gentle command of 'steady' can adopt a quieter pace.

Typically the horse appears to find that the entrance gate to the lunge area has a 'magnetic' effect! Thus the horse hurries round that part of the circle which heads towards the gate and then dawdles when heading away from the gate. A good lunger will quickly notice such things and by quiet movement will anticipate and counteract them

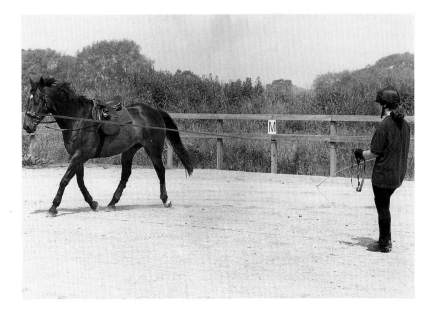

Fig. 11.6 Handler in the neutral position.

though this may not be apparent to an observer. If the horse pulls outwards, which may happen if the horse is over-fresh or badly trained, then it is helpful to lunge in an enclosed place. This may be the corner of the field or at the end of a school. In severe cases the open side can be enclosed with some jump poles on large oil drums or other temporary fencing. Such provisions should soon become unnecessary as the horse's manners improve.

On the other hand some horses charge inwards; the procedure is to stand your ground or even advance towards the horse with the lash of the whip looping towards the horse's barrel. If the lunger backs away then the horse has taken control and started to train the lunger. Commonly the horse will cut corners or fall in on the circle; in this case the whip should be pointed and, if necessary, flicked in the direction of the horse's shoulder. Sometimes a horse behaves like a hooligan and then it is necessary to attach the side reins straight away as clearly the horse is neither going to stretch down or relax, and the side reins will aid control.

When the horse has walked calmly for a few minutes on the left rein (anticlockwise), he should be sent round on the right rein (clockwise). The procedure is first to halt the horse out on the circle. He must not turn in and if he does he should be made to walk on again in the original direction. The command is a low and drawn out 'and whoa' accompanied by gentle vibration on the lunge line. If the horse does not halt, shorten the rein and bring him to a standstill. Firmly and consistently repeat this until he is obedient to the voice. When the horse is halted the lunger tucks the whip under their elbow, pointing to the rear, and walks towards the horse taking in the coils of line so that it does not hang slack or, worse still, touch the floor. Then, taking the horse on a short line, he is led round or across the circle to face the other way. Proceeding as before, the horse is sent round at a relaxed walk.

The time spent on the lunge will depend on the horse's stage of training, fitness and the type of work on the lunge; some purists like to see a horse walking for 20 minutes before trotting, but at least five minutes is a good aim. Having walked well on both reins, the horse can be given the sharp, quick command 'and trot'. If he does not respond at once a touch of the whip will serve to remind him. A crack of the whip takes only a flick of the wrist and can be useful and effective; however, care must be taken if other horses are close lest they too respond. The point is that the command should be said clearly and sharply but only once and the horse must obey instantly. Good lungeing makes the horse a better ride by enhancing obedience.

After the horse has trotted on both reins he can be halted and have the side reins fitted; initially these should be fairly long. The light pressure of the side reins on the bit may tend to shorten the horse's stride and so a little click of the tongue, a flick of the whip plus a sideways step to put the lunger a little behind the horse may be used selectively to maintain the quality of the movement. In trot the horse should put his hind feet into the prints left by the forefeet (Fig. 11.7). The trot circle should be at least 15 m (16 yd) in diameter.

Most lungeing for exercise is carried out at the working trot; this is a purposeful gait, not rushed but with a spring in the step. The side reins are shortened after a while as the horse is asked to accept a contact with the bit. In order to do this he must relax the jaw and flex the neck at the poll. He should also engage the hindquarters so that the hind legs step more actively under the body. However, he must not drop the contact with the bit by ducking the nose towards the chest so that the face makes a line behind the vertical. From time to time it is a good idea for the trainer or an experienced person to come and watch the lungeing so that bad practices do not creep in. When turning the horse round while he is still wearing side reins, lead the horse forwards in a small half circle; do not turn him on the spot.

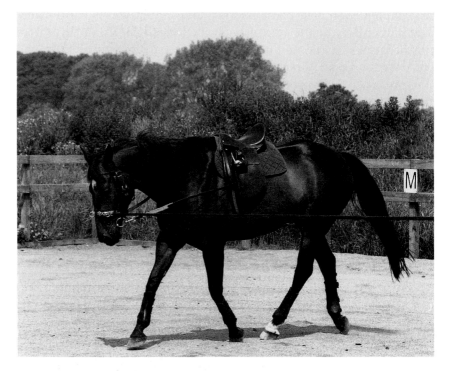

Fig. 11.7 A horse working happily on the lunge in trot.

Within the trot it is useful sometimes to ask the horse to do a few
lengthened strides. The easiest way to achieve this is to select a point of
the circle where there is a straight fence on the outside. Then with the
lunger running just a few steps parallel to the horse, he can be
encouraged to lengthen his stride before turning away from the fence
back onto the circle. Later it may be possible to produce lengthened
strides on the circle, but it is not an essential requirement to be able to
do so.

When the horse has worked calmly yet with good activity at the trot
on both reins he can be asked to canter. Experience will show the best
length of side reins in order to allow the horse to move freely forward
yet assist control and produce the round outline of the well-engaged
horse (one that is using his hindquarters to propel himself forward
actively). Sometimes, particularly in canter, the horse goes faster than
intended; in such cases the lunger should never resort to roughness.
The lunge line attached to the horse's nose has considerable leverage
and so a hefty yank could cause damage to the horse. The procedure if
the horse refuses to obey the voice commands of 'steady' or 'trot' is to

reduce the length of line fairly swiftly and bring the horse to a halt. Then impose discipline with walk to halt to walk transitions before proceeding to faster paces again.

In the canter it is particularly important that the circle is large enough; 20 m (22 yd) across is ideal so a lunge line of 10 m (11 yd) is required and for a fresh horse it should be longer. If the horse is to be cantered on the lunge the ground should not be deep or slippery as a poor surface can result in the horse knocking himself, losing confidence or losing the quality of the action. As in all lungeing, it is important that there is always a light, even tension on the lunge line. You should not have a tug-of-war or a slack line. Control of the spare coils of line is a skill needing practice and lack of good line discipline will result in the lunger either tripping over spare line or having line wound round the hand which could result in a nasty accident.

Practice for lungers

Lunge beginners can practice with the line attached to a fence post, letting it out, gathering it in, passing it into the other hand and so on; it is essential that the lunger never fails to have all the line under control and available as necessary. Even in practice, gloves must always be worn so that it is only natural to handle a lunge line when wearing gloves.

Similarly beginners must practise handling the lunge whip. Typically the whip is about 2 m (6 ft 6 in) long and the thong with lash an additional 3 m (9 ft 8 in). With the thong twisted round the whip it must be carried pointing behind the lunger; it must be brought quietly into the usable position and then tucked out of the way, pointing to the rear again when adjusting the side reins or turning the horse onto the other rein. The whip must not be laid on the floor in case it is trodden on; also, the lunger is in a vulnerable position and not in control when bending to pick it up. In use the whip rarely has to touch the horse, but such a delicate flick needs to be practised.

More advanced work

Trainers schooling horses on the lunge may sometimes shorten the inside side rein, but this is not usual when lungeing horses for exercise.

Similarly, trainers may usefully jump horses on the lunge; this is done without side reins and is an advanced skill.

In some cases an ill-disciplined or exuberant horse will go too fast or its hindquarters will keep flying outwards; in such a case a second lunge line is taken from the cavesson, round the hindquarters and so to the lunger's other hand. Great care has to be taken to prevent this line riding up under the horse's tail or slipping to the ground; this too is a form of exercise which is only suitable for those who are more experienced.

In long-reining there is a line to each bit ring and the lines either run through terrets on a roller or pad, or through rings on either side of a roller, and back to the lunger. Long-reining can be carried out using circles (Fig. 11.8) or straight lines (Fig. 11.9). Unless done with great care and skill the horse may tend to come behind the bit, that is drop the bit by bending the neck too much, tucking the nose into the chest, so that the face makes a line behind the vertical, and not go forwards with sufficient impulsion. Long-reining is a useful and enjoyable advanced skill.

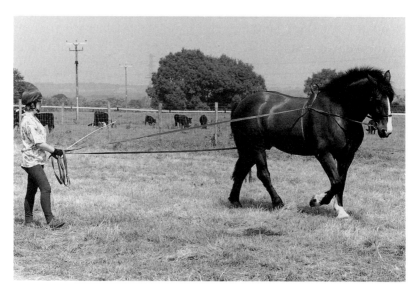

Fig. 11.8 Long reining on a circle.

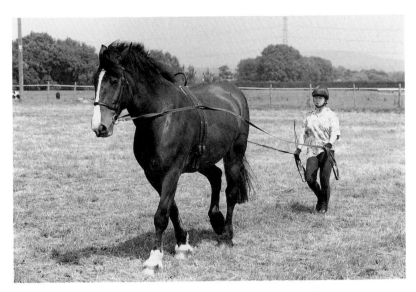

Fig. 11.9 Long reining on a straight line.

Part III
Horse Care in Action

12 Care of the Hunter

Getting the hunter fit

A fit horse is one that can do the work that is required of it without becoming overtired or overstressed. Getting a horse fit requires a mixture of correct work, feeding and health care. Regardless of the type of horse, the idea of the fitness programme is to improve the horse's ability to tolerate work by gradually increasing his workload and energy intake in a slow, steady progression.

The traditional methods of getting horses fit have developed from getting hunters fit from grass. Traditionally, hunters are brought up from grass at the beginning of August, allowing three months to get them hunting fit – equivalent to one-day-event fitness or 20-mile-distance ride fitness – before the Opening Meet in November. This three month period can be split into three four-week blocks: preliminary walking and trotting work, development work and fast work.

Bringing the hunter up from grass

After the hunting season the hunter will be roughed off and have a complete rest to allow him to unwind mentally and physically. The event horse has his break in the winter. The routine for bringing an unfit horse up from grass follows the same basic pattern, although there may be differences from yard to yard.

- *Vaccinations* – if the horse did not have the annual vaccination boosters before his holiday they should be given before starting any work. The horse will need seven days with no more than light work after vaccination to minimize the risk of any adverse reaction.
- *Teeth* – the vet or horse dentist should check the horse's teeth for sharp edges before the horse comes back into work and again six months later.
- *Worming* – a worming programme should be planned, with horses

being wormed when they are first brought in, and then every four-to-six weeks.

- *Shoeing* – horses must be shod all round once road work starts; a heavier set of shoes will last longer during this initial fittening period. The horse should be shod every four-to-six weeks.
- *Equipment* – the tack should have been stored in good condition at the end of last season. Check the stitching and restuff the saddle if necessary. Hunters can get very fat and soft during their summer break and so a thick numnah and a girth sleeve are a good idea to prevent rubbing and absorb sweat. The numnah and girth sleeve must be washed regularly. Salt water or methylated spirit can be applied to vulnerable areas on the horse to harden up the skin. Many people exercise horses in front boots plus knee boots when on the road; back boots can also be used if the horse's action makes them necessary.
- *Turning out* – the horse will benefit from being turned out for a few hours every day; this will help him unwind and stay sane. He has been accustomed to being out for most of the day and if part of the routine is a daily turn-out he is unlikely to have too wild a fling and gallop about. In the summer, horses should be protected from flies; otherwise they may become very frustrated and actually start to lose condition. Some people turn the horses out at night, exercise them early in the morning and keep them in during the day to avoid flies. This 'half and half' system is much better both physically and mentally for the horse than suddenly bringing him into work and stabling him full-time.
- *Feeding* – if the horse has not been receiving any concentrate feed, a small feed of a low energy food such as horse and pony cubes may be fed in the field the week before he is brought up. This will help his digestive system adjust to the feed he will be getting once stabled.
- *Trimming and bathing* – the horse will have his mane, tail, heels and whiskers trimmed, depending on individual preference. If the weather is mild he can be washed to help rid the coat of parasites, grease and scurf.
- *Preparation of the stable* – prior to the horse being brought back into work the stable should have been cleared of bedding, well scrubbed and then disinfected. Every so often the walls may need painting or treating with wood preservative. Hay and feed should be ordered and equipment such as buckets, clippers, etc. checked to ensure they are in sound working order.

Preliminary work

The preliminary work exercises the horse slowly for increasing lengths of time to tone up the muscles, tendons and ligaments and to harden the soft horse's skin. The initial walking and trotting work is very important.

Weeks 1 and 2: walking

The hunter is likely to have spent about four months in the field and may be rather fat and very unfit. This means that the work must progress slowly and steadily, starting with 20–30 minutes walking a day, building up to an hour by the end of the first week and two hours by the end of the second week. A horse walker can be used to do some of the walking work, or the horse can be led from another horse. Remember that this does not accustom the back muscles to carrying a rider and the girth region stays soft. Ideally the horse should be walked on the roads for up to two hours a day for four weeks and never less than two weeks – the longer the holiday the more road work is needed.

The horse must be carefully checked every day for rubs, galls and injuries. Girths and numnahs must be brushed after use and washed regularly to prevent them irritating the horse's skin.

Weeks 3 and 4: trotting

After at least two weeks walking work, trotting can be introduced; initially the trot should only be for a couple of minutes at a time, building up over the next few weeks to 15 minutes in total.

Development work

The next four weeks involve development work – the introduction of canter work so that the heart and lungs become accustomed to exercise. This builds up the horse's stamina while the muscles continue to strengthen and adapt to the work the horse is being given. The ground chosen for the first canter should be flat and not soft or dotted with potholes. The fresh horse may want to buck and gallop so be prepared for this – ask for canter quietly and keep the horse's head up. If the horse is known to be strong make sure that he is in suitable tack.

Canter work should be slow and steady initially and gradually increased so that by the end of the sixth week (mid-September) three or four periods of steady cantering a day can be included in the work. The horse should now be ready to go autumn hunting one or two mornings a week. Initially the horse should not stay out too long; it is very easy to start early and then stay out until lunch-time and find you have been out for four or five hours. Although you may not have been galloping and jumping, remember that just carrying a rider for a long time will be tiring to the semi-fit horse.

Fast work

The horse will need clipping as soon as his winter coat has grown adequately.

The hunter is rarely given any fast work during his exercise programme as October hunting usually provides enough cantering and the occasional short gallop (or 'pipe-opener') to prepare the horse for the Opening Meet. It is wise to school the hunter over cross-country fences once or twice before taking him hunting. It has been five or six months since he last jumped and it is a good idea to remind him about jumping. If you do not hunt in the autumn the horse will need to follow the programme outlined in the next chapter for the Novice event horse.

During the season

Throughout the hunting season days of sport will be interspersed with days of exercise. The exercise will vary depending on how hard the horse is working. A Hunt horse may do one or two hard days hunting a week. This will keep the horse fit and no more than 60–90 minutes walking with a little trotting will be needed on exercise days. Sunday is likely to be a rest day but rather than stand in his box the horse should be walked out in hand and allowed to graze for 10–15 minutes. This will help reduce the risk of azoturia.

A subscriber's (Hunt member's) horse may only hunt one day a week, that day being considerably less arduous than the Hunt horse's day. The subscriber's horse should have a short walk the day after hunting (usually a Sunday) and possibly a day off midweek when he should be turned out or walked in hand for 10–15 minutes. The remaining four days the horse should have 60–90 minutes of exercise including trotting and cantering. This horse may also benefit from a short gallop the day before hunting to clear his wind and prepare for the next day's galloping.

All horses vary in the amount of exercise they need to keep them in peak condition depending on how much hunting they are doing, their temperament and type. A hunter correctly worked and fed should stay in tiptop condition for the whole of the hunting season.

Roughing off

At the end of the season (March–April) the hunter is usually roughed off and turned out to grass for the long summer's rest. A clipped, corn-fed horse should not suddenly be turned out at this time of the year when the weather is cold, wet and unpredictable; the horse should be gradually 'let down'. Exercise should be reduced and at the same time the concentrate ration should be decreased and the amount of hay increased. As the weather gets warmer the number or weight of rugs should be reduced and the horse turned out for a greater length of time every day. Once the paddocks have dried up sufficiently to allow the horse to stay out all day he can stop being exercised and have his shoes removed. If the feet are likely to crack and spilt it may be necessary to leave the front shoes on. By the end of April or beginning of May the horse should be able to stay out day and night. A horse roughed off rapidly and turned out too soon tends to lose condition which may take a long time to recover.

During June and July flies can bother the horse, so any field should have adequate shelter. Alternatively the horse can be brought in during the heat of the day. The horse's feet must be regularly trimmed, he should be wormed every four-to-six weeks and checked daily for injury. The field must also be regularly checked for hazards that may injure the horse.

Feeding the hunter

As with feeding any horse it is a mistake to generalize and each horse must be fed as an individual and according to the amount of work done. A horse hunting two long days a week has widely differing requirements from a horse doing a short day once a week. However, the following points should be remembered:

- The horse must be fed to maintain condition for a long season. Traditionally boiled barley and linseed are fed; they are palatable feeds which help maintain the condition of horses that are working hard.
- The hours the horse spends out of the stable with a rider on his back are just as tiring as galloping and jumping.
- The hunter does not need to be as disciplined as the eventer or dressage horse; it does not matter too much if he starts the day a little fresh so long as he is still going at the end of the day – providing that the rider can cope!

- Feed should be reduced the day before a rest day. Traditionally the hunter receives a bran mash on the evening before his day off, its laxative effect helping to prevent azoturia.
- Tired horses tend to lose their appetite so it is better to feed smaller amounts of a high energy feed (performance cubes or cereals) rather than large amounts of a lower energy feed (horse and pony cubes).
- Succulents will tempt the shy feeder.

Care of the horse during the hunting season

The day before hunting

It is essential to be properly organized; equipment should be gathered together, cleaned and made ready for the morning. The following list covers the majority of equipment needed for hunting:

- Plaiting kit
- Grooming kit
- Tack – check the stitching for wear and polish bit rings and stirrups if necessary
- Brushing boots and over-reach boots if worn
- Headcollar and rope
- Travelling equipment for the horse
- Haynet for the return journey
- Sweat rug for the return journey
- Full water carrier and bucket
- Human first-aid kit
- Equine first-aid kit to include a small bowl, scissors, cottonwool, crepe bandages, gamgee, salt, wound dressings and sprays, and ready-to-use poultice.

The horse should be thoroughly groomed and have his mane, tail, feet and any white socks washed. If the whiskers and bridle path (parts of the head where the bridle rests) are trimmed they should be tidied up.

The hunting morning

Work backwards from the time of the Meet to calculate the time you should arrive and thus the time you must leave home, start plaiting and doing all the rest of the morning routine tasks and finally the time you must set the alarm clock. The horse must be fed at least an hour before the expected loading up time.

Before leaving, the horse should be groomed, the feet oiled and a tail bandage put on. Any small cuts should be dressed with antiseptic cream to protect them during the day. In countries where mud fever is a problem the horse's legs and belly are sometimes wiped over with oil to stop mud getting into the pores of the skin.

Hunters often travel tacked up with the headcollar on over the bridle and a rug and roller or surcingle over the saddle. If the journey to the Meet is short the horse may not wear any protective travelling gear except for a tail bandage. For longer journeys it is preferable for the horse to be adequately protected and tacked up on arrival.

The vehicle should be parked about a mile from the Meet – the hack helps settle the horse. Ensure that all equipment is safely put away and the vehicle locked up before leaving it.

Care after hunting

On a dry day the horse should be walked the last mile back to the vehicle so that he is cool and dry on arrival. However, if it is raining it may be better to keep trotting so that he arrives ready to be loaded warm and wet rather than cold and wet.

The bridle can be replaced with a headcollar and the horse either loaded immediately or tied to a string loop on the side of the vehicle. If the vehicle is parked on a busy road, it is wet or the horse excited it is probably better to load him immediately. The saddle will have been on for a long time so either the girth can be loosened, the sweat rug and top rug placed on top and the horse travelled home with the saddle on, or the saddle can be removed and the area under the saddle patted briskly to help the circulation in the blood vessels under the saddle to return; sudden removal can cause scalded backs and pressure lumps. The horse can then be rugged up.

The horse can be offered a small drink of water (no more than a quarter of a bucket) and any obvious injuries attended to. Travelling gear can then be put on the horse and he can have another small drink before travelling home with his haynet.

On returning home

The routine followed varies between yards but the following guide-lines may prove useful.

(1)   Once the horse has been unloaded he can be taken to the stable, tied up beside a haynet, have the saddle and travelling gear removed and the rugs thrown back over him.

(2)   He can be offered water at regular intervals. If he drank a couple of times before being loaded he can have half a bucket of water, followed 15 minutes later by as much as he wants to drink. However, if he has not drunk all day he should be restricted to a quarter of a bucket every 15 minutes until his thirst is quenched. Very tired horses may appreciate water that has had the chill taken off it. Dehydrated horses can either be offered electrolytes in the feed or in a separate bucket of water. It is important that the horse drinks but does not gorge himself on water, risking colic.

(3)   Meanwhile the horse can have his feet picked out, shoes checked for soundness and legs checked for injuries such as thorns and cuts. He can then be cleaned. If he is dry the mud can be brushed off and sticky sweat marks sponged off with warm water. If the mud is wet some people prefer to leave it to dry and to brush it off in the morning while others wash it off immediately, either with a hose or sponge and warm water. If the horse is washed he should be towelled dry before being rugged up with dry rugs. Stable bandages will help support tired legs and dry wet ones. The tail should be washed and the plaits taken out. If the horse is very tired just make him clean enough to be comfortable and leave him to rest. Keep offering the horse water until his thirst is quenched.

(4)   The horse can now be left in peace with his haynet and a small feed.

(5)   The tack can be cleaned. Some yards wash the mud off now, leave the tack to dry and soap it the next day, while others clean it completely the same evening.

(6)   The horse may break out in a sweat. Check him every 15 minutes for cold, sweaty patches, restless behaviour, disturbed bedding or a reluctance to eat. If the signs are mild keep the horse warm by rubbing his ears until they are warm and walk him (if the weather is suitable) until he is dry and comfortable. If the horse does not respond or looks very distressed then veterinary help should be called.

(7)   Before leaving the horse, top up the water buckets. The horse should be checked later in the evening, given more water and hay as well as a late night feed.

The day after hunting

Providing that the horse has eaten up and looks well he can be fed and given hay as normal. Depending on the routine followed the previous night the horse may be clean or dirty. Any stable bandages should be removed and the legs carefully checked for heat, pain or swelling from cuts, thorns, knocks or strains. The rugs can be thrown back and the saddle and girth area checked for lumps or rubs. The horse can then be unrugged and trotted up in hand to check that he is sound; he may seem stiff initially but this should soon wear off. The rugs can then be thrown back over the horse while he is thoroughly cleaned, making sure that awkward areas such as between the hind legs and elbows are attended to. Once the horse is clean he can be exercised. The amount of exercise will depend on how hard he worked the day before; it is likely that 15–30 minutes' walk will be enough. The horse can then be returned to the stable and left in peace to recover from his exertions.

13 Care of the Competition Horse

Getting the competition horse fit

Bringing the competition or event horse up from grass and then getting him fit varies very little from the programme outlined in Chapter 12 for the hunter. The main differences are that, firstly, the event horse is being got fit in the winter prior to competing in the summer and, secondly, he needs to follow a more formal fast work plan in order to reach the desired level of fitness.

Bringing the competition horse up from grass

The event horse usually has a rest in the winter and is brought back into work in December or January ready for the first event in March or April. This means that he is generally stabled at night and is already being fed concentrates so that unlike the hunter his system does not need to become accustomed to a completely different regime. He will also need clipping as soon as he comes into work; a blanket clip keeps his back warm during the preliminary work. He can have a hunter clip when he starts to do faster work.

Interval training

Interval training has become popular for training competition horses. It consists of giving a horse a period of canter followed by a brief interval of walk during which the horse is allowed to partially recover before being asked to work again. Interval training increases the horse's capacity for using oxygen to create energy; the point at which the horse runs up an oxygen debt is delayed as much as possible. This results in the horse being able to work for longer before fatigue sets in. The interval training workouts are fitted into the total training programme of the horse. (See also Appendix: Interval Training to Novice One-day-event Fitness: a Detailed 12-week Schedule.)

188

An essential part of the interval training regime is monitoring the horse's temperature, pulse and respiration (TPR) to gauge the horse's reaction to the work. Interval training cannot cut corners and the following factors must be considered before starting such a programme:

- The horse should be capable of 90 minutes walk and trot over rolling terrain without distress. The horse conditioned slowly and carefully will stay in peak condition longer than one pushed too fast in the early stages.
- It is essential to keep a notebook with a running record of the horse's response to the workout, allowing the programme to be adjusted accordingly.
- As in any form of training the rider must be alert to any change in the horse's attitude, appetite, coat, droppings, appearance, muscle tone, etc.

During interval training the horse is cantered at a predetermined speed for a certain time. After this the horse is pulled up and the pulse and/or respiration rates are recorded immediately. The horse is then walked for a set time and the rates recorded again. The difference between the two readings is the 'recovery rate' of the horse. This fast then slow work is repeated two or three times.

These workouts are repeated, usually every four days, and the pulse and respiration rates recorded at the same points; as the horse gets fitter he will recover faster from the work. Fitness is gradually built up by slowly increasing the total amount of work the horse is asked to do and by increasing the speed and/or length of the workout or using more demanding terrain. If the recovery rate is not good enough after a workout, the work should be adjusted so that the horse is never overstressed.

Points to remember

- Interval training must be monitored by pulse and respiration rate, not by time alone. It is the pulse rate immediately after the workout that shows how much stress the horse has been subjected to, and the recovery rate that shows how fit he is.
- If the pulse and respiration have not returned to normal within 20 minutes of completing the workout the horse has been overworked and the programme should be adapted accordingly.

- The respiration rate should not exceed the pulse rate; if it does stop work.
- Never complete the day's planned programme if the horse becomes distressed.
- On the other hand the horse must be stressed enough to stimulate the body systems to become better adapted to exercise. The heart rate must be raised above 100 beats per minute after work.
- The interval training programme should be planned backwards from the proposed date of the competition(s) so that workout days fall appropriately.
- Always warm up and cool down thoroughly before cantering, particularly if the horse has to travel in a lorry or trailer to the work area.

Preliminary work

The preliminary work is no different for the competition horse than for the hunter – they both need plenty of slow work at the beginning of the programme.

Weeks 1 and 2: walking

Not all riders allow their horses to become completely unfit; they may only give their horses a short holiday of two-to-four weeks, after which they are walked two or three times a week for up to an hour each time. This helps to maintain a basic level of fitness and to keep the tendons and bones strong. The risk of girth galls and sore backs is also lessened.

During preliminary work, ideally the horse should be walked on the roads for up to two hours a day for four weeks and never less than two weeks – the longer the holiday the more road work is needed. If the horse has been walked two or three times a week from the field, another two weeks on top should suffice once the horse has come in to be stabled. This work strengthens the horse and prepares him for the next stage. The walk should never be sloppy; it should be purposeful and with a good rein contact.

Weeks 3 and 4: trotting

After at least two weeks' walking work, trotting can be introduced; initially the trot should only be for a couple of minutes at a time, building up over the next couple of weeks to 15 minutes in total. If the trotting is done in an arena sharp turns and small circles must be avoided at this stage. Flat work or lungeing can be incorporated into the routine towards the end of the fourth week; this should be no more than 30 minutes before or after an hour's road work.

It is far better to underfeed than overfeed the horse with concentrates at this stage, but a good amount of hay (or a dust-free equivalent such as haylage) must be fed to prevent the stabled horse becoming bored.

Development work (weeks 5 and 6)

Development work involves the introduction of canter work and suppling exercises so that the heart and lungs become accustomed to stronger exercise, building up the horse's stamina while the muscles continue to strengthen and adapt to the work the horse is being given.

The initial canter work may be done in a schooling environment where horses often respect their riders more than in an open space. The horse should be cantered for two-to-three minutes at 400 m per minute to start with, bringing the horse back to walk through trot. These little bouts of canter should be built up so that by the end of two weeks the horse is cantering for a total of nine-to-ten minutes split into three or four sessions. The horse should always be walked for two-to-five minutes after each canter.

During week 5 or 6, jumping can be introduced into the programme starting with pole work, grid work and small jumps in the school. This can be incorporated into the schooling programme so that by the end of the second month the novice horse should have done a small local show jumping class or two.

Discipline work (weeks 8–12)

The third period of the fitness programme is even more specialized; the power and athleticism of the dressage horse (Fig. 13.1) and show jumper (Fig. 13.2) are developed further, while the racehorse and the event horse are given fast work. Some horses, for example ridden show horses, do not need speed, power or athleticism but should continue to build up body, skin and coat condition and become more highly trained.

Now interval training can start in earnest. Canter work is repeated every fourth day, building the sessions up minute by minute. The day after a canter session should be less stressful with a hack or some gentle schooling. Over the next two weeks the sessions are built up so that the horse can do three lots of five minute canters at 400 mpm, with 3 minutes' walking in between.

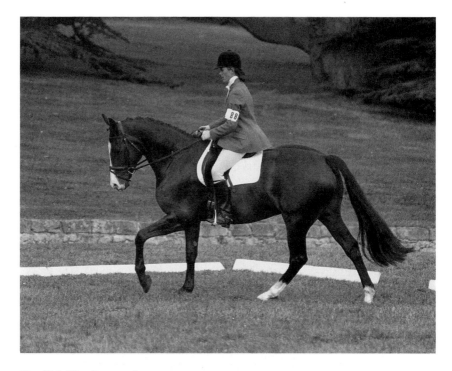

Fig. 13.1 The dressage horse.

By now the horse will have been stabled about ten weeks. Road work continues each day; it can form a useful warming up and/or cooling down period. Show jumping, cross-country and dressage schooling all continue in a balanced programme.

The final two weeks (weeks 10–12)
The first horse trial can be planned for week 12; on a couple of occasions, the last minute of the last canter can be increased to a speed of 500 mpm.

Table 13.1 shows a sample workout. The heart rate after the third canter should drop below 100 beats per minute after ten minutes walking. All horses are individuals and must be treated as such. Tables are merely a guideline and do not allow for lost shoes, heavy-going or lazy horses. The real skill in training lies in the ability to design programmes for individual horses and to recognize the need to adapt the programme without hindering the horse's progress. The same programme may take up to two weeks longer with a different horse.

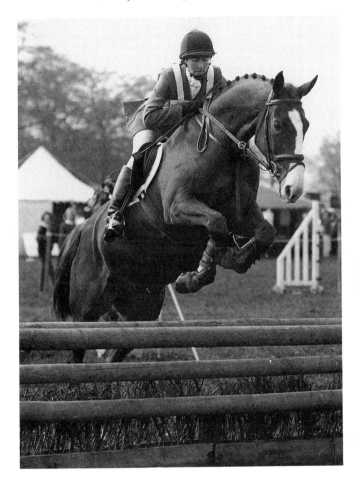

Fig. 13.2 The show jumper.

Roughing off

Once the competition season has finished the horse may be roughed off and turned out to grass for a holiday. The horse's work is cut down or stopped and he is turned out in the field for an increasing amount of time during the day, regardless of the weather. Gradually the number of rugs worn is reduced and the ratio of forage to concentrates increased. The shoes may be removed or left on according to the state of the horse's feet. Hind shoes may be removed if there is a danger of horses kicking each other. The horses should have their feet checked regularly while at grass and also should be wormed.

Table 13.1 Interval training to novice one-day-event fitness.

20 minutes warm-up		
Canter 1:	5 minutes @ 400 mpm	
	trot 30 seconds	
	walk 3 minutes	
Canter 2:	4 minutes @ 400 mpm	
	1 minute @ 500 mpm	
	trot 30 seconds–1 minute	
	walk 3 minutes	
Canter 3:	4 minutes @ 400 mpm	
	1 minute @ 500 mpm building up to 550 mpm	
	trot 1–2 minutes	
	walk at least 20 minutes.	

Feeding the competition horse

The competition or event horse has to be fit enough to gallop and jump at speed and yet disciplined enough to perform dressage and show jumping; this has led to many event riders trying to keep their horses happy both mentally and physically by feeding as few concentrates as possible and turning their horses out in the field every day. The three-day-event horse may have a very rigorous training programme and yet only compete in a few events on the run up to the main competition before being turned away, while the lower level horse may compete once a week throughout the long event season. These horses have widely differing feed requirements.

Prior to the event do not be tempted to change the horse's ration. Some people reduce or omit the sugar beet pulp from the feed before the event, while others would only do this on the morning of a cross-country event. If the horse frets away from home, reduce the quantity of concentrate food and use high energy palatable ingredients such as milk pellets and flaked maize. Generally speaking, however, it is better not to alter the horse's feed too much; you may just cause problems.

A three-day-event horse should have a concentrate feed no less than four hours before the start time of the first phase of the cross country day. If competing in the afternoon he could also be given a small haynet. If the horse has had free access to fresh water there is no reason why he should have his water bucket taken away before competing – why should he suddenly decide to have a huge drink?

A novice event horse could munch on a haynet while being plaited on the morning of the competition. If he is competing early he should not receive any bulk feed while travelling until after his cross-country event. If he is competing later he could have a small haynet while travelling. Depending on your competing times, he may be able to have a concentrate feed between the dressage and the show jumping, providing that there is at least two hours digestion time. He should be offered water frequently throughout the day and allowed to wash his mouth out between the show jumping and the cross-country, even if they are very close together.

The fluid and electrolyte balance is very important and the horse must be watched for signs of dehydration. If a pinch of skin on the neck or shoulder lingers after it has been released and the horse has a gaunt tucked-up appearance he may well be dehydrated – this can limit the next day's performance severely. Ensure that the horse drinks and provide electrolytes in the food or water.

Colic can be a problem after severe exertion, and the intestines must be kept moving. Once the horse is cool and his thirst has been quenched he may appreciate a small bran mash, with his normal feed later on. Tired horses are easily overfaced by a large feed, but dividing the normal feed in two and feeding it at intervals may overcome this.

After the competition the horse's appetite will indicate how tired he is. Until he is eating normally, he has not really recovered from his exertions and should be allowed plenty of rest. Hacks and grazing in hand will help the horse relax and recover.

Care of the horse during the competition season

The week before the competition
This is the time for those finishing touches. The mane and tail should be tidied up and the horse clipped if necessary. All tack and equipment must be examined thoroughly and repaired or replaced; any items missing from your checklist must be purchased and ensure that any medications are not out-of-date. The horse should be shod with stud holes as necessary and the farrier asked to check that the horse's spare set of shoes still fit correctly. The numnahs, boots and rugs, etc. that are being taken to the competition should be clean and in good repair.

The day before the competition
If staying overnight before or after the competition it is essential to be properly organized; clean equipment should be gathered together and

packed. The following list gives the general requirements for most situations:

- Stable tools, muck skip and muck sack
- Shavings or paper bedding
- Two haynets
- Two water buckets and full water carrier
- Feed bowl
- Pre-packed concentrate feeds clearly labelled, for example, 'Monday lunch'
- Soaked sugar beet pulp if fed
- Hay or haylage
- Supplements, for example, electrolytes
- Grooming kit including extra sponges, towels, sweat scraper and hoof oil
- Fly spray
- Plaiting kit
- Spare set of shoes, studs and stud fitting kit
- Tack cleaning kit
- Spare rugs and blankets
- Sweat sheets or coolers
- Waterproof rugs
- Stable bandages and gamgee or wraps
- Passport/vaccination certificate
- Rule book and details of entry
- Equipment for all those going on the trip (food, clothing, toiletries, money, etc.).

Other essential items include:

- Tack – depending on the horse and competition
- Bandages, brushing boots, over-reach boots plus spares
- Spare girth, leathers, irons and reins
- Spare headcollar and rope
- Hole punch
- Lungeing equipment
- Travelling equipment for the horse
- Human first-aid kit
- Equine first-aid kit to include a small bowl, scissors, cottonwool, crepe bandages, gamgee, salt, wound dressings and sprays, ready-to-use poultice and leg coolant.

The horse should be thoroughly groomed; if the weather permits it may be possible to bathe him, and you will need to wash the mane, tail and any white socks. If the whiskers and bridle path are trimmed a last trim will prevent a designer-stubble look.

Packing the vehicle

Equipment should be listed and ticked off as loaded; this will avoid vital items being overlooked. Containers as simple as plastic washing baskets will make loading and unloading easier, but they should not be too large or too heavy as this makes handling tricky. Containers should have an easily-read list of contents so that items can be located quickly. Filled water containers and buckets should be packed so that they are easy to get at during the journey for watering the horse.

At the competition

Find out when the class starts or your specific start times so that you know in advance the time your horse is expected to compete. Work backwards from this time to calculate the time you should arrive at the showground and thus the time you must leave home, start plaiting and doing all the rest of the morning routine tasks, and finally the time you must set the alarm clock.

The horse must be fed at least an hour before the expected loading up time. Allow extra time for delays in the journey and about 45 minutes-to-an-hour to get yourself organized and the horse settled and tacked up before he needs to be ridden. If you have a cross-country course to walk allow yourself an hour to do this plus 10 minutes to walk the show-jumping course.

Once at the competition ground, park where the ground is as level as possible, and if the weather is warm try to find some shade. If you have help and the horse has had a long journey he should be quietly unloaded and walked in hand; letting him graze will help relax him. Meanwhile you can go and declare for the class, pick up your number and find out where everything is. The next step is to brush the horse over; he will have been thoroughly groomed at home and should only need the finishing touches such as hoof oil, quarter marks and the last shaving taking out of his tail. If the competition is on grass the horse may be fitted with studs to give him more grip. The type of stud used will depend on the state of the going with pointed studs being used on hard ground and square studs on soft ground. The horse is now ready to be tacked up, mounted and warmed up.

Overnight stays

If staying overnight at a showground or racecourse all the horse's vaccination papers should be up-to-date and ready to show the officials. Before putting the horse into the stable, which may be temporary or permanent, carry out a few checks:

- Clean out contaminated or mouldy bedding.
- Wash out the manger, disinfect and then wash it again.
- Clean out the automatic drinker if present.
- Check that the lights work and are out of reach of the horse.
- Check that glass-covered windows are safe and out of reach of the horse.
- Ensure that there are no sharp edges or projections which may cut the horse.
- The door must be strong with secure latches and bolts.

Once the horse has been unloaded and has had a walk to stretch his legs he can go into the stable for a roll. After being offered a drink, he will benefit from a small haynet to munch on so that by the time he is offered a feed he is relaxed enough to eat it. Even if the horse does not have a late night feed he should be checked last thing to see that he has settled in this strange environment and is not too warm or too cold.

Care after the competition

After the horse has finished an arduous competition he will have a higher temperature, pulse and respiration rates and it is important to bring these body systems back to normal as quickly as possible.

(1) Immediately after the horse has stopped the rider should dismount and loosen the girth; it is important to keep the horse moving so that the circulating blood cools the muscles. After 5 minutes walking, the horse can have the tack removed and a cooler or sweat rug put on and walking continued. If the saddle has been on for a long time, it should be left in place for about 10 minutes to allow the circulation in the blood vessels under the saddle to return; sudden removal can cause scalded backs and pressure lumps.

(2) As soon as the horse stops blowing hard he can have a few sips of water. Until the horse is cool and his thirst quenched he should be given water little and often; as a guide allow five swallows of water for every 50 m walked.

(3)   The pulse and respiration rates of a fit horse that has not been over stressed should return to comfortable levels within 15 minutes and the horse should be checked every 15 minutes thereafter until the values return to normal, which should be within an hour of completing exercise.

(4)   Once the pulse and respiration are within comfortable levels the horse should be stood in a sheltered place, out of the sun on a hot day and out of the wind on a cool day, and washed down. The lower legs, inside the legs, the head and belly should be sponged, but the large muscle masses of the back and quarters must be avoided as sudden cooling can send them into spasm.

(5)   During untacking and sponging, the horse must be checked for injury; once he has recovered, these areas can be cleaned and dressed. The horse should also be jogged for a few yards to check for soundness while he is recovering.

(6)   Once the horse has cooled completely he can have a nibble of grass or a small haynet while you attend to his legs. The leg treatment will vary according to personal preference, but after strenuous effort it is a good idea to apply a cold dressing to constrict the blood vessels and soothe any bruising and inflammation that may be present. A clay or cooling gel dressing can be used and applied thickly down the back of the leg from the knee to below the fetlock joint, and then covered in dampened newspaper, tinfoil, clingfilm or plastic with gamgee and a stable bandage applied over the top.

(7)   Although the skin and surface muscles are now cool, the horse may break out in a sweat. Check the horse every 15 minutes for cold, sweaty patches, restless behaviour, disturbed bedding or a reluctance to eat. If the signs are mild keep the horse warm and walk him until he is dry and comfortable. If the horse does not respond or looks very distressed then veterinary help should be called.

Welfare of the competition horse

Whatever type of equestrian sport is being followed it is vital that the competition horse is looked after in the best way possible. The following points are included in a Code of Conduct which has been drawn up by the Federation Equestre Internationale (FEI) in conjunction with The International League for the Protection of Horses (ILPH) and the British Equestrian Federation (BEF).

- In all equestrian sports the welfare of the horse must be considered paramount.
- The well-being of the horse is more important than performance in a competition; horses must not be exploited to satisfy a sponsor or team.
- The pressure to compete must not result in the misuse of medication.
- The highest standards of feeding, health and stable management must be maintained.
- The horse must be travelled with adequate ventilation, feeding, watering and rest periods.
- The horse's rider or driver must be fit and competent.
- No training method should cause pain, injury or distress.

14   Care of the Leisure Horse

A large number of horses are kept by riding schools or private owners as leisure animals. They are not kept to take part in a specific equestrian sport, but provide enjoyment to their riders hacking and taking part in a variety of competitions and club activities. These horses may compete in dressage, hunter trials, show jumping and showing classes as well as doing the odd day's hunting and the occasional sponsored ride or team chase.

The majority of texts are written for the professional full-time horse person. However, many horse owners are in other full-time work; indeed, they need to work in order to pay the bills associated with keeping a horse! Fitting a horse in around your life and commitments is not easy and must be planned so that neither the horse nor the family are neglected.

The right horse for the job

Selecting the right horse is the first step on the way to a happy partnership. Owning a leisure horse is supposed to be fun; unfortunately it can turn out to be a nightmare if the horse is unsuitable. The ideal horse is a 'can't go wrong' character; he should be rugged, amenable and a pleasure to own and look after. There are guidelines that will help in choosing the right horse:

- A cob or pony cross is likely to be sensible and easy to feed.
- The horse does not need to be much higher than 15.2 hh. Providing that he is sturdy and has plenty of bone, that is the circumference of the leg below the knee is adequate for the size of horse, he should be able to carry any person's weight. Ability is not related to size and a 15.2 can do anything that a 16.2 can do.
- Smaller horses tend to be more sound and easier to look after. Large often means trouble.

- Avoid Thoroughbreds as they tend to need plenty of work every day and are not suited to being amenable at the weekend having done little all week.
- Avoid buying a young horse unless you have enough time and expertise to train the horse.
- When choosing a horse take a knowledgeable friend with you.
- Before buying the horse have it vetted; the expense is well justified.

Keeping the horse in the stable

The horse is not designed to be kept in a stable; he does not have enough space to move around in, there is very little air space, the air only changes slowly resulting in a stuffy atmosphere and he has no real physical contact with other horses. All in all it is a totally artificial lifestyle. However, stabling horses is very convenient for us: we can feed and exercise them, keep them warm and dry, prevent them being kicked or bitten by other horses and keep more animals on a small piece of land. After all, most people cannot afford to buy a paddock but we can afford to rent a stable.

It is important that the stable is an adequate size: for example, 3.5 m² (12 ft²) is a minimum size for a 16 h horse. Further details regarding the size of stables can be found in *Horse and Stable Management*. The stable should also be well ventilated; in most ready-made boxes the window and door are on the same side and as a result the open top half of the door often blocks the window and there is no movement of air through the stable. While the horse must not stand in a draught it is useful to have a window or gap below the eaves on the opposite side from the door to ensure that the air within the box changes regularly, creating a healthy environment. There should also be an exit for air in the ridge of the roof; this allows the warm air to escape from the stable as it rises and effectively 'sucks' air in through the open top half of the door.

Keeping the horse at grass

There are many advantages in keeping the horse at grass: it is a natural system; less straw and hay are used; less time is spent on routine management; and the horse need not be ridden because it will exercise itself. However, there are disadvantages: the horse may become too fat in the summer; he may be wet and muddy in the winter; he still needs to be caught and checked over every day; supplementary feeding will be necessary in the winter and in the summer where there is insufficient grass.

It is easier to operate a 'combined system' where the horse spends part of the day at grass and the rest of the time in the stable. In the summer the horse can be stabled during the day to protect him from the flies. In the winter the horse may be stabled at night or brought in well in advance of being ridden to give him time to dry.

A variation of the traditional system of in at night, out by day which, although expensive initially, offers many advantages of the paddock without the mess, is that of the shelter/stable with a free-draining sand yard attached. The horse can be shut in the stable at night and then allowed access to the yard during the day. This way the horse has a little more exercise, plenty of fresh air and a more natural environment.

Horses working from grass in the winter can be given a trace or blanket clip. This makes grooming easier and allows the horse to work without undue sweating. A clipped horse will need a New Zealand rug. An unclipped horse can be turned out without a rug, but the heavy winter coat will take a long time to dry before the horse can be tacked up. The horse will dry quite quickly if put in the stable with a thatch of straw on his back, lightly covered with a cut-open light-weight hessian sack held in place with a loosely-fastened surcingle. After half-an-hour or so the worst of the mud can be brushed off with a dandy brush. If the horse's girth and saddle area are not free of mud there is a risk that the horse's skin will be rubbed and sore after riding.

After work the wet horse should not be left in the stable. If he is to remain stabled, he should be thatched in order to aid drying. If the horse is to be turned out, this should be done straight away so that he can roll and keep on the move.

Keeping the leisure horse fit

The leisure horse is unlikely to undergo a formal fitness programme. The work done will vary according to the rider's ability, facilities and preference, but the horse will rarely be more than half fit, having undergone the equivalent of the preliminary and development stages outlined earlier.

If the horse is going to compete in hunter trials or to go hunting it is important that some faster work is done prior to the event. This faster work may take the form of going round a farm ride, for example, and cantering where possible. This also gives the rider the opportunity to pull their stirrups up and get themselves fit for riding short at the same time. Alternatively, the canter work could be done in the arena – the horse will not be able to go fast but there is no reason why the rider cannot shorten the stirrups, adopt a forward seat and do, say, three three-minute canters. Both horse and rider may be competent at jumping but unless they are both fit problems are likely to arise towards the end of the course.

Feeding the leisure horse

It must always be borne in mind that the domesticated horse is being given a diet that is quite different from the one he is designed to cope with. In the wild he would graze and browse a high fibre diet for up to 16 hours a day. In an effort to keep the horse slim and athletic we cut down the fibre, reduce the eating time and add highly digestible concentrates to the ration.

It is easy to overestimate the feed requirements of a horse that is working for an hour a day, hacking or doing school work. Just because we have worked hard riding the horse does not mean that the horse has worked equally hard. Many behavioural problems as well as health problems are caused by overfeeding. The golden rules for safe, economical and effective feeding are:

- Feed simply.
- Feed plenty of roughage and as few concentrates as possible.
- Buy the best quality hay you can afford.

Feeding a low energy, high fibre compound feed such as horse and pony cubes along with dust- and mould-free hay should be all that the healthy leisure horse needs. If he is inclined to bolt his feed, chaff can be added to slow him down and make him chew the feed more thoroughly. There should be no need to add a supplement or 'a bit of this and a bit of that' to the feed as it will only unbalance the ration that the equine nutritionist has created. In the winter the horse will appreciate carrots in the feed. Horses that are allergic to the dust and fungal spores found in hay may need to have their hay soaked or they can be fed a dust-free alternative such as haylage.

If the horse is turned out onto reasonable grazing in the summer he may only need feed and hay if he is brought in at night. The amount of feed will depend on the quantity and quality of the grazing available. If the horse is inclined to become fat try to turn him out on sparse grazing so that he has to work hard for each mouthful of grass. Keeping him in and starving him during the day will only encourage gorging at night.

Caring for the leisure horse after exercise

Although the leisure horse may not work hard in the accepted sense he will often be hot and tired after exercise. As he is only half-fit he will find the exercise just as strenuous as the fit horse in an arduous competition. See the section 'Care after the competition' in Chapter 13.

Selecting a system of management

The important thing with a leisure horse is to set up a system which maximises the pleasure of ownership, whether it is your own stable and paddock or a 'do-it-yourself' livery. Take good local advice to ensure that the system and facilities will meet your needs and provide you and your horse with the greatest enjoyment.

Appendix: Interval Training to Novice One-day-event Fitness: A Detailed 12-week Schedule

Throughout the fitness programme the horse should be turned out for a couple of hours whenever possible, particularly on rest days. All hacks should be for a minimum of one hour.

Week 1
    Day 1: 20 minute walk
    Day 2: 30 minute walk
    Day 3: 40 minute walk
    Day 4: 50 minute walk
    Day 5: 60 minute walk
    Day 6: 60 minute walk
    Day 7: Rest day

Week 2
    Day 1: 1 hour 10 minute walk
    Day 2: 1 hour 20 minute walk
    Day 3: 1 hour 30 minute walk
    Day 4: 1 hour 40 minute walk
    Day 5: 1 hour 50 minute walk
    Day 6: 2 hour walk
    Day 7: Rest day

Week 3
    Day 1: 2 hour hack including one 400 m (1 minute 50 seconds) trot
    Day 2: 2 hour hack including two 400 m trots
    Day 3: 2 hour hack including three 400 m trots
    Day 4: 1 hour 30 minute hack including two 800 m (3 minute 40 seconds) trots
    Day 5: 1 hour 30 minute hack including three 800 m trots; check recovery

Day 6: 1 hour 15 minute hack including two 1100 m (5 minute) trots

Day 7: Rest day

Week 4

Day 1: 1 hour 30 minute hack including three 5 minute trots; check recovery

Day 2: As Day 1

Day 3: 1 hour walk plus 20 minutes schooling

Day 4: As Day 1

Day 5: 1 hour walk plus 20 minutes schooling

Day 6: As Day 1

Day 7: Rest day

Week 5

Day 1: 1 hour 30 minute hack including three 5 minute trots and one 1 minute canter (400 m at 400 mpm); check recovery. The canter work may be done in the school.

Day 2: 1 hour walk plus 20 minutes schooling, including pole work

Day 3: 1 hour walk plus 30 minutes schooling

Day 4: 1 hour 30 minute hack including three 5 minute trots and two 1 minute canters; check recovery

Day 5: 1 hour walk plus 30 minutes schooling, including small jumps

Day 6: 1 hour 30 minute hack including three 5 minute trots and three 1 minute canters; check recovery. Alternatively, a dressage competition

Day 7: Rest day

Week 6

Day 1: 1 hour 30 minute hack including three 5 minute trots and two 2 minute canters (800 m at 400 mpm); check recovery

Day 2: 1 hour walk plus 40 minutes schooling, including pole work

Day 3: 1 hour walk plus 40 minutes schooling, including small jumps

Day 4: 1 hour 30 minute hack including three 5 minute trots and three 2 minute canters; check recovery

Day 5: 1 hour walk plus 40 minutes schooling

Day 6: 1 hour 30 minute hack including three 5 minute trots and two 3 minute canters (1200 m at 400 mpm); check recovery. Alternatively, a small show-jumping competition

Day 7: Rest day

Week 7

Interval training begins in earnest and the 4-day schedule is adhered to as far as possible.

Day 1: Hack
Day 2: 1 hour hack plus 40 minutes schooling
Day 3: 1 hour hack plus 45 minutes schooling and jumping
Day 4: 45 minute hack plus three 3 minute canters at 400 mpm with 3 minute walk between; check recovery
Day 5: Hack
Day 6: 1 hour hack plus 40 minutes schooling
Day 7: A dressage or show jumping competition

Week 8

Day 1: 45 minute hack plus one 3 minute canter and two 4 minute canters at 400 mpm with 3 minute walk between; check recovery
Day 2: Rest day
Day 3: 1 hour hack plus 40 minutes schooling
Day 4: 1 hour hack plus 45 minutes schooling and jumping
Day 5: 45 minute hack plus three 4 minute canters at 400 mpm with 3 minute walk between; check recovery
Day 6: Hack
Day 7: 1 hour hack plus 40 minutes schooling

Week 9

Day 1: 1 hour hack plus 45 minutes schooling and jumping
Day 2: 45 minute hack plus two 4 minute canters and one 5 minute canter at 400 mpm with 3 minute walk between; check recovery
Day 3: Rest day
Day 4: 1 hour hack plus 40 minutes schooling
Day 5: 1 hour hack plus 45 minutes schooling and jumping
Day 6: 45 minute hack plus one 4 minute canter and two 5 minute canters at 400 mpm with 3 minute walk between; check recovery
Day 7: Hack

Week 10

Day 1: 1 hour hack plus 40 minutes schooling

Day 2: 1 hour hack plus 45 minutes schooling and jumping

Day 3: 45 minute hack plus three 5 minute canters at 400 mpm with 3 minute walk between; check recovery

Day 4: Rest day

Day 5: 1 hour hack plus 40 minutes schooling

Day 6: 1 hour hack plus 45 minutes schooling and jumping

Day 7: Cross-country schooling to replace canter work

Week 11

Day 1: Hack

Day 2: 1 hour hack plus 40 minutes schooling

Day 3: 1 hour hack plus 45 minutes schooling and jumping

Day 4: 45 minute hack plus one 5 minute canter at 400 mpm, two 4 minute canters at 400 mpm finishing with one 1 minute canter at 500 mpm with 3 minute walk between; check recovery

Day 5: Rest day

Day 6: 1 hour hack plus 40 minutes schooling

Day 7: 1 hour hack plus 45 minutes schooling and jumping

Week 12

Day 1: Hack

Day 2: 45 minute hack plus one 5 minute canter at 400 mpm, one 4 minute canter at 400 mpm plus one 1 minute canter at 500 mpm, one 4 minute canter at 400 mpm plus one 1 minute canter at 550 mpm with 3 minute walk between; check recovery

Day 3: Hack

Day 4: 1 hour hack plus 40 minutes schooling

Day 5: 1 hour hack plus 45 minutes schooling and jumping

Day 6: FIRST HORSE TRIALS

Day 7: Rest day

Index